Fundamental Aspects of Community Nursing

Fundamental Aspects of Community Nursing

Second Edition

MARIE DREYER
SUSAN HATTINGH
MARGUERITE LOCK

OXFORD
UNIVERSITY PRESS

OXFORD
UNIVERSITY PRESS

Great Clarendon Street, Oxford OX2 6DP

Oxford University Press is a department of the University of Oxford.
It furthers the University's objective of excellence in research, scholarship, and education by publishing worldwide in

Oxford New York

Athens Auckland Bangkok Bogotá Buenos Aires Calcutta Cape Town Chennai Dar es Salaam Delhi Florence Hong Kong Istanbul Karachi Kuala Lumpur Madrid Melbourne Mexico City Mumbai Nairobi Paris São Paulo Shanghai Singapore Taipei Tokyo Toronto Warsaw

with associated companies in Berlin Ibadan

Oxford is a registered trade mark of Oxford University Press in the UK and certain other countries

Published in South Africa
by Oxford University Press Southern Africa, Cape Town

Fundamental Aspects of Community Nursing
ISBN 0 19 571996 4

Previously published by Southern Book Publishers (Pty) Ltd (1868640175)
First edition 1993
Second edition 1997
Reprinted 1998, 2000

Cover design by Collage Graphics

Published by Oxford University Press Southern Africa
PO Box 12119, N1 City, 7463, Cape Town, South Africa

Set in 10 on 12 pt Palatino Roman
Typesetting and reproduction by PG&A, Ottery, Cape
Printed and bound by NBD, Drukkery Street, Goodwood, Western Cape

Contents

Acknowledgements

We are indebted to several people who were instrumental in the formulation and production of this book. The most important are the students who used the first edition. Their feedback was invaluable in the writing of this second edition.

We also wish to thank the following people:

- Jean-Jeanette Kotze for her endless patience in typing and re-typing the manuscript and teaching us how to use the word processor;
- Our colleagues in the Department of Nursing Science who never failed to believe in us and who encouraged and motivated us to write this book;
- Leanne Martini and Eloise Wessels of ITP for their professionalism and support at a crucial stage in the development of the manuscript;
- Sarie Human for her constructive criticism and valuable contribution to the contents of the book;
- Our families and friends for their support and understanding.

Most importantly, we thank God for giving us the courage and ability to write this book.

1 Philosophical views on community nursing and community health care

MARIE DREYER

CHAPTER OBJECTIVES

After reading this chapter, the student should be able to:

- describe the concepts discussed in this chapter;
- identify the characteristics of a science;
- outline the scientific characteristics of nursing and community nursing;
- describe a philosophy of health;
- formulate a philosophy of community nursing;
- identify the basic principles of ethics; and
- discuss ethical dilemmas that may occur in community nursing.

1.1 INTRODUCTION

The scientific foundations of nursing are often debated by people from other disciplines as well as within the profession itself. In this debate there is considerable confusion about whether nursing is a science or not.

In the past nursing relied to a great extent on the theories of other disciplines such as sociology. It is only in recent years that nurses started to do independent research and developed their own theories and body of knowledge.

To defend the scientific grounding of the profession, it is essential that nurses should keep abreast of new developments and views about the scientific merits of nursing. Brink (1992:12) states that to be able meaningfully to participate in such debates or to defend their views when challenged, it is essential for nurses to have an understanding of nursing science and how it relates to the large body of science. In this chapter the focus will be on the views of some nurse theorists and other experts regarding the scientific basis of nursing and community nursing. Aspects such as the philosophy of community health and community nursing as well as certain ethical principles will also be outlined.

1.2 WHAT IS A SCIENCE?

The question is often asked whether or not nursing is a science. Before that question can be answered, let us examine what is meant by a "science".

Various perspectives on the nature of scientific knowledge, the meaning of the term science and the characteristics of a science can be traced in scientific literature. According to logical empiricists the term science refers to a product – a set of statements that forms the body of knowledge and is frequently referred to as traditional science or pure science. Historicists, on the other hand, understand science as the processes of human behaviour or science practice, such as experimenting and compiling data, and they view science as a process of understanding human behaviour.

Rogers in Barrett (1990:6) describes science as an organised abstract system – a synthesis of facts and ideas, or an organised body of abstract knowledge arrived at by scientific research and logical analysis. Brink (1992:12) indicates that the nature of science is a controversial issue and that conceptualisations vary according to the world view or philosophical orientation of the scientist. From the various views it can be deduced that science is both a product and a process, with the product representing the ever-growing and ever-changing accumulated knowledge of a discipline, i.e. the body of knowledge. The process refers to the methods of gathering and collating the data from which the body of knowledge evolves.

Although there are many approaches to the definition of a "science", certain basic common features can be identified:

- the observation and description of phenomena in real life;
- the use of scientific methods and tools to gather data;
- an empirical verification of statements and assumptions;
- a theoretical grounding and logical reasoning;
- the synthesis, classification and organisation of facts; and
- a specific scientific language or terminology.

1.3 WHAT IS A DISCIPLINE?

Brink (1992:13) indicates that it is only logical also to define the concept of discipline when dealing with the meaning of the concept of science because most of the definitions are, according to Moody (1990:18), given within the context of the discipline from which they arise. According to Mellish (1982:139), a discipline can be defined as a branch of instruction or teaching and the discipline of nursing refers to the instruction or teaching of the art and science of nursing, which is a unique, dynamic discipline based on the physical and biological as well as social sciences.

Each discipline has a central focus that influences the perspective of its field, but no discipline is totally independent. Consensus has been reached amongst some nursing theorists that the central focus in nursing is the person, the environment and health. According to Marriner-Tomey (1989:15), one goal of science is the identification of truths or facts about the subject matter of a discipline, i.e. the phenomena of interest in that specific discipline.

1.4 IS NURSING A SCIENCE?

Having established what is meant by a "science" and a "discipline" and having determined the characteristics of a science, we now turn to the scientific basis of nursing and examine the various opinions which have been expressed on the subject.

In the past nursing was considered as the art of caring for the sick and nurturing the healthy development of young and old alike. The emphasis was on the functions or activities carried out by nurses and most definitions of nursing focused on caring for and assisting the sick individual. Until recently the art of nursing was viewed entirely in terms of compassion, humanity and the ideals of service. In other words, most descriptions focused on the skills or activities and not on the application of nursing theories or knowledge.

A more contemporary definition of nursing is provided by Griffith-Kenney and Christensen (1986:10), who state that nursing is an art and science that applies intellectual, interpersonal and technical skills throughout the nursing process to assist clients in achieving their maximum health potential.

Furthermore, until the 1960s, nursing was viewed as an applied science because it relied on the theories and knowledge of the physical, behavioural and humanistic sciences. Subsequently, nurse leaders have become more aware of the need to develop and clearly delineate a theoretical base and body of knowledge specific to nursing, which could distinguish it from other disciplines. As nursing moved into higher education and increasing numbers of nurses graduated and conducted research in nursing, theories, concepts and terminology specific to nursing were developed (Ference in Malinski 1986:35).

The knowledge base changed and expanded rapidly and "by the 1970s the profession viewed nursing as a scientific discipline evolving towards a theory-based practice that focuses on the client" (Griffith-Kenney and Christensen 1986:4).

The views of various nurse theorists and leaders in nursing are given in the nursing literature. Some of these will be highlighted in this section. Central to most of these definitions are the concepts of science and art.

According to Yurra and Walsh (1978:16), science implies knowledge or conceptualisation, while art presupposes action. The goal of the science of nursing is the understanding of the phenomena of nursing, while the art is the application of the knowledge in practice.

The following definitions and descriptions reveal the views of some nurse theorists on nursing as a science.

Ziegler *et al.* (1986:14) maintain that nursing is an applied science that utilises theories from other disciplines to understand the phenomena that are of concern to nursing, as well as those theories specific to nursing.

Rogers, a nurse theorist (in Barrett 1990), describes nursing as a science and an art. She argues that the term "nursing", which signifies a learned profession, is a noun and not a verb. She further argues that the noun "nursing" specifies an organised body of knowledge specific to its central purpose, and that the creative use of this body of knowledge is the art of nursing.

According to Rogers, contemporary nurse scientists define distinctive knowledge bases for nursing a person. Barrett (1990:31) maintains that "science-based practice is the use of substantive nursing knowledge, developed through logical analysis and quantitative and qualitative modes of inquiry".

Smith (1981:2), citing Hokey (1973), indicates that nursing is the art of applying nursing science. The South African Nursing Council describes nursing science as a human clinical health science that constitutes the body of knowledge for the practice of persons who are enrolled or registered as nurses or midwives under the Nursing Act. Within the parameters of nursing philosophy and ethics, it is concerned with the development of knowledge for diagnosis, treatment and personalised health care.

According to Yurra and Walsh (1978:16), "the art and science of nursing are integral parts of the nursing process". The systematic assessment of the client/patient, problem identification, scientific planning and implementation of nursing action takes place within a scientific framework.

According to these descriptions, a specific body of knowledge is regarded as necessary for nursing practice.

Hein and Nicholson (1986:130) maintain that without a science of nursing, the art of nursing would be impossible.

From contemporary nursing literature, it is clear that nursing is a functional science based on theories from other sciences as well as on specific nursing theories. It is also clear that the discipline of nursing uses the general principles of the scientific method, namely that of gathering knowledge, synthesising facts, logical reasoning, predicting and explaining phenomena in the field of nursing. Nursing science in this context thus refers to the body of knowledge on which nursing practice is based as well as the methodologies used to gain the knowledge.

1.5 IS COMMUNITY NURSING A SCIENCE?

Before it can be established whether community nursing meets the criteria of a science, the unique features of this discipline must be explored. Community nursing is defined as follows by Hanlon in Clark (1984:32):

> . . . a field of specialisation within both professional nursing and the broad area of organised public health practice. It utilises the philosophy, content and methods of public health and the knowledge and skills of professional nursing. It is responsible for the provision of nursing services on a family centred basis

for individuals and groups at home, at work, at school and in public health centres.

Spradley (1990:65) describes community nursing as a field of practice that synthesises knowledge and skills from nursing and community health and applies them towards the promotion of optimal health for the total community. She further indicates that community nursing is not a setting-based but a knowledge-based practice and that this discipline is based on community health science as well as on nursing science. Thus the foundation of community health primarily lies in disease prevention and health promotion. In other words, a registered nurse with additional qualifications in community nursing science can work in a hospital or in the community (setting-based), but specific knowledge is required for a registered nurse to be a community nurse (knowledge-based).

This branch of nursing requires a thorough knowledge of the discipline of community nursing.

According to the American Nursing Association, community nursing is more than just generic nursing carried out in non-hospital settings, but it is a synthesis of nursing practice and public health practice applied to promoting and preserving the health of populations.

Clark (1992) identified certain unique elements specific to community nursing:

- *Health orientation:* emphasis on health promotion and disease prevention rather than the curing of illnesses.
- *Population focus:* emphasis on population groups rather than on individuals or families.
- *Autonomy:* greater control over health care decisions by both nurse and client than in other settings.
- *Continuity:* provision of care on a continuing basis rather than on a short-term, episodic basis.
- *Collaboration:* interaction between nurse and client as equals; greater opportunity for collaboration with other segments of society.
- *Interactivity:* greater awareness of the interaction between health and a variety of other factors.
- *Public accountability:* accountability to society for the health of the general population.
- *Sphere of intimacy:* greater awareness of the reality of clients' lives and situations than is true for other areas of nursing.

From the aforementioned characteristics, it is clear that community nursing science is a specialised area of nursing. Its main purpose is to provide nursing care to population groups or families and individuals outside the hospital environment. It is primarily concerned with the prevention of disease and the promotion of health.

Community nursing synthesises the practice and knowledge of community health science with the theories of professional nursing science to provide preventive, promotive, curative and rehabilitative health care to communities.

It can be argued that community nursing is a science because nursing theories form the foundation for practical application, and the knowledge and skills of community nursing are those of professional nursing practice. Community nursing utilises the concepts, knowledge and skills of community health science to become a speciality with its own distinctive body of knowledge.

1.6 A PHILOSOPHY OF COMMUNITY NURSING

A philosophy is regarded as a certain view of and attitude towards life that explains the origin, nature, purpose and existence of life and that directs behaviour and activity. It is a statement that reflects the values, goals or opinions and beliefs of an individual, community or discipline. Thus we believe that statements associated with nursing practice contribute to the philosophy of the discipline of nursing.

According to Burgess and Ragland (1983:9), a philosophy helps to clarify and establish one's orientation to life or to a particular aspect of life as well as to explain one's beliefs and values to other people.

It determines the principles according to which a person lives, his or her ideals and the way in which the person strives to fulfil these ideals. It is not concerned with the scientific process of experimentation, observation, and description – it concentrates on the goal and meaning of life.

A philosophy can be described as a statement of beliefs that reflects our values and orientation, which in turn form the basis for our practice and professional activities. A philosophy of community nursing should be based on the philosophical views of nursing as well as on the philosophical views of health and health care within a specific community.

Central to all nursing is caring, which comprises interaction between the nurse and the client or patient, producing therapeutic results in the persons who are served. The basis for this caring process is a philosophy of nursing within a specific community or culture that gives direction and determines the attitudes of nurses and the way they interact with their patients/clients as well as their colleagues, the public and other professionals. Marriner-Tomey (1989:16) maintains that the prevailing philosophy of a discipline is the one shared by the greatest number of members in terms of accepting the beliefs, values, goals, and opinions of the philosophy.

Community nurses should be orientated to study and to understand the philosophical baseline of nursing as described in nursing literature, as well as the philosophy of health and health care. With this knowledge in mind, a community nurse can formulate her own community nursing philosophy.

Without a philosophy it is impossible to provide quality community nursing care.

According to Searle (1986:259), "the personal and professional philosophies of the individual in any category of nursing determine how she will develop her own expertise and how she will use this expertise to meet the human need for health care". A philosophy will thus guide the community nurse in her interpersonal relations, social behaviour and the application of her therapeutic skills.

The community nurse, like all other categories of nurses, must remember that the purpose of nursing is the welfare of her patients and that nursing is in fact a moral art. According to Hein *et al.* (1986:130), it is a moral art because it involves other human beings and our relationships with them, as well as the promotion of what is generally regarded as "good health".

According to Jones (1991:267), the philosophy of humanitarianism that demands that health care delivery must be available to all people is extending the role and functions of the nurse. This requires adjustment of the philosophy of care so that the community nurse can provide a comprehensive health care service that integrates preventive, promotive, curative and rehabilitative health care to achieve the goal of optimal health for all.

The philosophy of community nurses thus forms an integral part of community nursing science. It is based on a certain view of the individual, the community, health and nursing, and it influences the community nurse's behaviour towards families, groups and collaborators. A philosophy determines how the community nurse behaves and functions within the framework of a system for community health care delivery.

The community nurse is involved in complex long-term personal interactions, direct practice and professional as well as political issues that directly affect the community. It is therefore important that the community nurse should have a sound philosophy of her own. This will enable her to support and help families in their own environment and to resolve problems and value-related conflicts.

1.7 A PHILOSOPHY OF COMMUNITY HEALTH AND COMMUNITY HEALTH CARE DELIVERY

The philosophy of communities or individuals about good health varies in nature according to their knowledge of health and illness as well as their cultural differences.

A philosophy of health flows from the sense of national responsibility and the consciousness of a community of the value of good health.

In developed as well as in developing countries the World Health Organisation's definition of health as a "state of complete physical, mental and social well-being and not merely the absence of disease and infirmity" is accepted as the core philosophical view of health. Most literature emphasises the fact that health encompasses the well-being of body, mind and spirit, and the harmonious integration of a person with himself, society and the environment.

This implies that the nurse should provide holistic care for her patients, and that health care delivery should meet the needs of the individual as a whole. Holistic health is defined by Edelman and Mandle (1990:8) as "the integration of the mind, body, spirit and environment". According to the Collins Dictionary (1991:342), holism means the "treatment of any subject as a whole integrated system, especially in medicine the consideration of the complete person". Health care delivery should therefore cater for a person as a whole and to be able to achieve this, a philosophy of comprehensive health care to improve the quality of the physical, mental and social health of individuals, families and communities is accepted by most countries.

Community health practitioners believe that the attainment of optimal health for all citizens is of great importance and that the following aspects are inherent in any philosophy for health care delivery:

- health care delivery must be comprehensive to provide for the health needs of all age groups from before birth to death;
- all members of a family must understand that their state of health is their own responsibility;
- the community as a whole must participate in the prevention of disease, the prolonging of life and the promotion of physical as well as mental health through organised team efforts;
- health care practitioners should assist and teach individuals and families to take responsibility for their own health and to become involved in the planning and provision of health care;
- the primary objective must be to keep people healthy – good health must be stressed; and
- health development is an integral part of social development.

Inherent in modern health care philosophies is the idea that primary health care is the key to the attainment of optimum levels of health for all people in situations where resources are very limited. This implies that health care delivery should be accessible, affordable and acceptable to a specific community.

The philosophy of primary health care is based on three pillars, namely:

- commitment to greater justice and equity in health-resource allocation;
- adherence to the principle of the right of people to be involved in significant decisions concerning their health services, i.e. community involvement in health; and
- the acceptance of the need for the medical profession to collaborate with other sectors.

The philosophy of health in a specific community is expressed in the measures taken by the community to promote good health and to prevent disease.

The above beliefs and pillars form the basis for the philosophy of health care delivery in South Africa. Community nurses form part of the health care system and all endeavour to provide a comprehensive health care service to cater for all people from birth until death. They are committed to develop and utilise the existing and potential knowledge, skills and resources of communities and to interact and collaborate on a continuous basis with all the major role players in the community.

1.8 THE ETHICS OF NURSING AND ETHICAL DILEMMAS IN THE COMMUNITY HEALTH FIELD

Closely related to a philosophy of nursing are the ethical principles and codes of the nursing profession. Ethics in nursing refers to the codes and professional conduct of the registered nurse. According to these codes, the professional nurse must be accountable and credible. This implies that the nurse must always act in such a way as to promote and safeguard the well-being of her patients/clients and that she is responsible for her own actions and omissions.

Ethics can be described as values or standards that govern the behaviour of a group - they determine whether the actions taken are right or wrong. Community nurses are concerned with both medical and community health ethics (Clark 1992:265). Ethical behaviour in the field of health care delivery is based on the principles of beneficence, autonomy, self-determination and justice or equity:

- Beneficence involves promoting the interests of clients. It focuses on positive steps to be taken to prevent harm to a person, for example legislation to wear safety belts.
- Autonomy refers to the right of the individual to make his or her own decisions and choices. This also includes the right to confidentiality, privacy and the right to refuse treatment.
- Self-determination refers to the patient taking responsibility for his or her own state of health.
- Equity or justice involves the fair distribution of benefits, goods and services - it is based on the belief that all groups of people should be treated equally and that each person should receive a decent share of the goods and services available.

1.8.1 Approaches to making ethical decisions

In the process of making ethical decisions, the following should be kept in mind:

- Consequential decisions are based on the outcomes of actions. These decisions are the result of egoism, i.e. the decisions are based on how the outcome will affect oneself. Consequential decisions may also be based on utilitarianism, where the decision is taken on the basis of which action will cause the least harm, and on libertarianism where the decision will protect the right of the individual.

Ethical decisions made from a utilitarian perspective are based on the action that will achieve the most good or will cause the least harm for most people. For example, the community nurse may decide to discontinue her services to a client who is not benefitting from her care. Instead, she will provide care to those who will really benefit from such a service, which will be for the greater good for the whole community.

The principle of libertarianism is that of professional liberty, and ethical decisions made on this basis attempt to protect the right of the individual to achieve self-determination. Libertarian arguments are often used against legislation mandating immunisation against communicable diseases, for example, and against the compulsory use of helmets by motor-cyclists. According to Clark (1992:268), libertarianism claims that mandates like these supersede the principles of autonomy, self-determination or the right to choose to act in an unhealthy manner.

- Non-consequential decisions are based on duty and responsibility. In this case, the question whether an action is right or wrong is at issue. Non-consequential decisions also take into account the duties that may arise from contracts between people.

1.8.2 Ethical dilemmas in community nursing

The community nurse will experience many ethical conflicts in contemporary community health care and must be familiar with ethical principles and their application in certain situations. In these decisions the community nurse will be guided by her own personal values and norms, as well as the established ethical codes pertaining to the nursing profession. Ethics guide health care providers in determining the morally correct action in a given situation.

A knowledge of the ethical codes laid down and adhered to by the nursing profession is of great importance because the professional nurse is always responsible for her own actions and omissions. She must examine her own values to be able to make ethical decisions.

Ethical dilemmas arise when a choice has to be made between two unacceptable decisions. Decisions of this nature may cause conflict and feelings of guilt on the part of both the patient and the nurse. For example, when a mother is advised to have a therapeutic abortion, her feelings about terminating the pregnancy may cause a certain amount of conflict. The same applies to a nurse who has to assist a doctor with an abortion, or a community nurse who is faced with caring for a patient with AIDS. For ethical reasons and according to her professional codes of conduct, she cannot refuse, even though, in the case of the AIDS patient, she may be very much afraid of contracting the disease.

It is therefore the responsibility of the community nurse to advise and support her client in situations where value-related or conflicting decisions need to be made. She must inform her client regarding all the possible positive and negative aspects, thus enabling the client to make a well-informed decision. In making a nursing diagnosis where an ethical dilemma arises, the community nurse should consider the existence of such a dilemma as well as the possible value conflicts. The course of action can be selected after the values involved have been identified.

The community nurse is often in the unenviable position where she has to make conflicting decisions, for example whether or not to participate in a strike. On the one hand, she knows her responsibility towards her client/patient, but on the other hand she is threatened with possible harm to her family if she does not participate.

Ethical dilemmas may be inherent in numerous circumstances (Clark 1992:270–2):

- a person's right to health care and his or her right to make health-related decisions;
- the responsibility of society to provide health care for all citizens;
- the allocation of resources, for example, whether advanced technology, such as the facilities to perform heart transplants, should be made available when a great number of people do not have access to basic health care; and
- death and dying, for example, the wish of a terminally ill patient for euthanasia.

In the course of her duty the community nurse may be faced with many ethical dilemmas. For instance, the question may arise who should take responsibility for the health of a person who chooses to act in an unhealthy manner. Similarly, she may be faced with a decision on where the responsibility of health care practitioners ends and where individual responsibility begins. In all situations, a thorough knowledge of the ethical principles of her profession, together with her personal values and norms, will assist her in making morally correct decisions.

1.9 SUMMARY

In this chapter, an overview is given of arguments on the question whether nursing is a science. The views of various authors are noted and it is clear that nursing can be considered as a science with its own body of knowledge on which the practice is based. Furthermore, the development of a philosophy of community nursing as well as of health and community health care delivery is discussed. Aspects closely related to the philosophy of nursing, namely nursing ethics and ethical dilemmas in the community health field, are described.

QUESTIONS

1. Formulate a philosophy of community nursing.
2. What do you understand by the term "ethical dilemma"?
3. List arguments that can prove the scientific foundation of nursing and community nursing.

FURTHER READING

Barrett, E.A.M. 1990. *Visions of Rogers' science-based nursing*. USA: National League for Nursing.

Burgess, W. & Ragland, E.C. 1983. *Community health nursing. Philosophy, process, practice*. Norwalk, Connecticut: Appleton-Century-Croft.

Clark, M.J. 1992. *Health care in the community*. Norwalk, Connecticut: Appleton & Lange.

BIBLIOGRAPHY

Barrett, E.A.M. 1990. *Visions of Rogers' science-based nursing*. USA: National League for Nursing.

Brink, H. 1992. "The science of nursing: current issues and dilemmas." *Curationis*, Vol. 15, No. 2.

Burgess, W. & Ragland, E.C. 1983. *Community health nursing. Philosophy, process, practice*. Norwalk, Connecticut: Appleton-Century-Croft.

Clark, M.J. 1992. *Health care in the community*. Norwalk, Connecticut: Appleton & Lange.

Clark, M.J.D. 1984. *Community health care for today and tomorrow*. Reston: Prentice-Hall.

Collins English Dictionary. 1991. Glasgow: HarperCollins.

Conway, M.E. 1985. "Toward greater specificity in defining nursing's metaparadigm." *Advances in nursing science*. 7(4), 73–81.

Edelman, C.L. & Mandle, C.L. 1990. *Health promotion throughout the lifespan*. St Louis: Mosby.

Griffith-Kenney, J.W. & Christensen, P.J. 1986. *Nursing process. Application of theories, frameworks and models*. St Louis: Mosby.

Hein, E.C. & Nicholson, M.J. 1986. *Contemporary leadership behavior: selected readings*. Boston: Little, Brown and Company.

Jones, K. 1991. *Sociology of health and illness*. Cape Town: Juta.

Malinski, V.M. 1986. *Explorations on Martha Rogers' science of unitary human beings*. Norwalk, Connecticut: Appleton-Century-Croft.

Marriner-Tomey, A. 1989. *Nursing theorists and their work*. 2nd edition. St Louis: Mosby.

Mellish, J.M. 1982. *Etos van verpleegkunde*. Durban: Butterworths.

Moody, L.E. 1990. *Advancing Nursing Science through Research*. Vol. 1. Newbury: Sage Publications.

Searle, C. 1986. *Professional practice: a South-African nursing perspective.* Durban: Butterworths.

Spradley, B.W. 1990. *Community health nursing. Concepts and practice.* Glenview: Scott, Foresman.

Smith, J.P. 1981. *Nursing science in nursing practice.* London: Butterworths.

Yurra, H. & Walsh, M.P. 1978. *The nursing process: assessing, planning, implementing, evaluating*. New York: Appleton-Century-Crofts.

Ziegler, S.M. *et al.* 1986. *Nursing process, diagnosis, nursing knowledge.* Norwalk Connecticut: Appleton-Century-Crofts.

2 The scientific method of nursing applied in community nursing

MARIE DREYER

CHAPTER OBJECTIVES

After reading this chapter, the student should be able to:

- describe the concepts that appear in this chapter;
- describe the various elements of the nursing process;
- understand the relevance of the nursing process to community-orientated nursing practice;
- develop a nursing care plan; and
- evaluate the nursing intervention and care.

2.1 INTRODUCTION

In this chapter the various steps or elements of the nursing process, as they apply to community nursing practice, will be outlined. The emphasis will be on the assessment of the client (either an individual, a family or a community); the formulation of a community nursing plan or programme; the implementation and evaluation of the plan; the recording of all data and information collected; and the diagnosis, treatment and care of clients.

2.2 THE NURSING PROCESS

According to Clark (1984:179), the nursing process is an organised scheme of nursing intervention that is comprised of four distinct steps: assessment, planning, implementation and evaluation. Although records are kept throughout, a fifth step – recording – is added to the nursing process in South Africa. This is necessary because nurses are responsible for their own actions and omissions. In this context records could serve as decisive documents in any enquiries into negligence.

The number of steps in the nursing process may vary according to the views of different theorists. Nursing literature in general places increasing emphasis on interaction (i.e. communication and interpersonal relationships) as a component of the nursing process because it is an essential element in any nursing activity. A community nurse should be competent in interpersonal skills to be able to communicate with her clients and to interview them in various situations.

Spradley (1990:213) regards the nursing process as one of the essential dynamics in community nursing practice, as it provides the active driving force for change. According to Spradley, the following three characteristics emphasise the importance of this tool in community nursing:

- the problem-solving process that addresses community health problems;
- the management process that requires analysis, decision making, planning and controlling, and evaluation; and
- the change process that works to improve health-related systems and the way people behave within these systems.

Whereas the nursing process focuses on the individual patient in the hospital setting, in community nursing practice the focus is on the three types of client, i.e. community, the family and the individual who receives the nursing care:

- *The community as a client:* Three types of community are identified, i.e. people living within a specific geographical area, people with the same interests and people with the same health problems or needs. The entire community is the focus and recipient of health care.
- *The individual as a client.* This is an individual within the community or family or workplace with a specific health care need. This may be a child, an adolescent, an adult or an aged person.
- *The family as a client:* This refers to a specific family within the community with a specific health care need.

Within the framework of the nursing process, scientific assessment, planning, implementation and evaluation of nursing care or intervention is outlined to ensure effective action through which the health of the community can be improved. A specific conceptual model can be selected to guide the community nurse through all the steps of the nursing process. In community nursing, Orem's model can be applied to aid the client, for example one with a self-care deficit.

In summary it can be said that the nursing process provides the methodology for scientific nursing care, as each step of the process ends in a product and all steps are interrelated.

It must, however, be emphasised that in community nursing practice there are certain key areas that require clarification. According to Burgess (1983), key phrases in the definition of the nursing process must be examined, such as: Who is the client? What does the client's problem signify in the community health care situation? It must be kept in mind that the client can be an individual, a family or a community, and that this client is involved in the planning and decision-making process.

Furthermore, community nursing focuses not only on problems, but also on the level of the client's wellness, his or her strengths and the risk factors

FIGURE 2.1: The interrelationship between the various elements of the nursing process

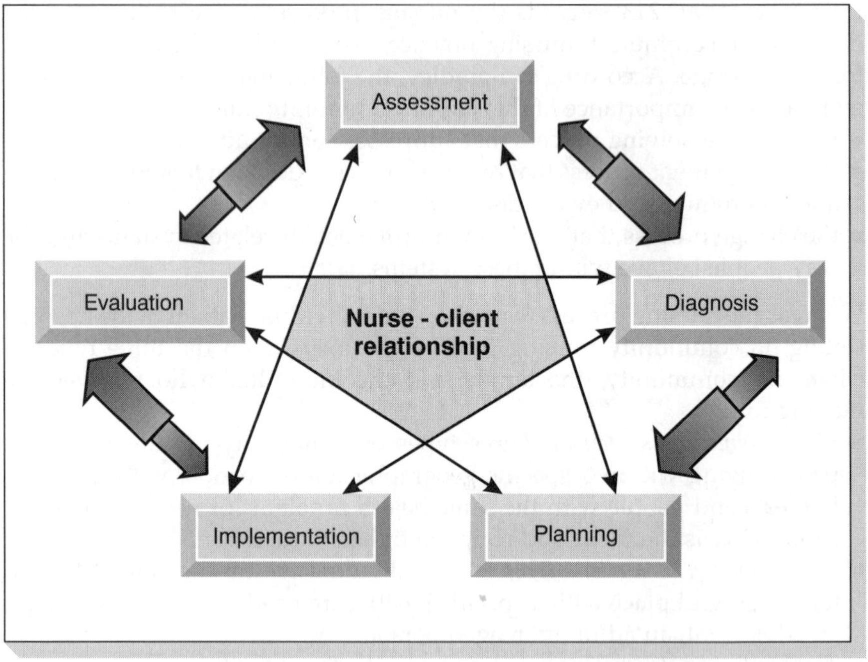

pertaining to his or her situation. The primary concern of community nursing is the prevention of disease and the promotion of good health.

2.3 THE FIVE STEPS OF THE NURSING PROCESS

2.3.1 Assessment

Assessment may be regarded as the most important step of the nursing process. Prior to any nursing action, the nurse must assess the client's situation and identify any problems requiring intervention. This is the first step and the data collected during this phase form the foundation of the nursing process. The nursing diagnosis is based on the interpretation of the collected data or identified problems.

Assessment can be described as an act of appraisal whereby the health status and needs of the client are judged as a basis on which to plan the action. Yurra and Walsh (1978:27) describe assessment as "the act of reviewing a situation for the purpose of diagnosing the client's problems". In community nursing, assessment can be described as the act of becoming acquainted with a community.

Burgess and Ragland (1983:47) indicate that the assessment phase consists of four nursing actions:

- the selection of data collection tools and data sources;
- the collection of data;
- the organisation and analysis of findings; and
- the formulation of a nursing diagnosis.

When an assessment is conducted, the nurse should, according to Ziegler *et al.* (1986:55):
- identify the client;
- identify the purpose of data collection;
- determine the data collection methods to be used;
- determine the sources to be used to collect data;
- collect objective as well as subjective data; and
- record the data in the data base.

The collected data may consist of one or a combination of the following:
- a family profile;
- a health history;
- a community profile; and
- a physical examination.

The assessment process will also depend on which nursing model has been chosen. If Orem's model is used, data regarding health deviations, self-care deficits and requisites should be collected (Ziegler *et al.* 1986:57).

The community nurse makes assessments that are more wideranging and more detailed than the nurse practising in other areas because she does not normally deal with life-threatening situations and has more time to collect data. For example, the assessment of families in their homes will be different from the process used in a hospital setting. It will take longer and will be more detailed.

The collection of data usually starts prior to the interview when the addresses of the people to be interviewed are noted and the nature of other sources (such as statistics) are studied. According to Clark (1984:203), data collection usually includes a health history, physical examination and appropriate screening. In the community health setting, an assessment of the individual, family or community should be health-orientated and the physical, sociological and emotional needs must be observed. The individual in the community health situation cannot be assessed in isolation because he or she is influenced by the environment and interpersonal relations with members of the family, as well as by variables in the community.

A community assessment can be carried out by using various data collection techniques such as interviews, questionnaires or observations. Research methods such as surveys, case studies or epidemiological studies are suitable for studying a community, family or an individual. Some of the major sources of information are health, vital and census statistics. Data collection depends to a large extent on communication, interviewing and observation skills. Data collection tools, too, must be reliable and valid. Primary as well as secondary sources can be used, for example interviews with consumers of health care and client records, or previous research reports. (Primary sources report original work, while secondary sources focus on other people's work. Research reports are a combination of primary and secondary sources.)

It is of extreme importance that a comprehensive, systematic assessment should be carried out that facilitates the diagnosis, decision-making and planning processes. When data are collected, consideration should be given to actual as well as potential needs, as this will influence decisions regarding actions and priorities (Spradley 1990:217).

After an analysis of the data that have been collected, a nursing diagnosis can be made.

Ziegler *et al.* (1986:43) describe a nursing diagnosis as "a statement of client response related to aetiology, that the nurse can independently diagnose and treat". Price (in Burgess & Ragland 1983:49) indicates that "a nursing diagnosis identifies an existing or potential health problem that nurses are qualified and licensed to treat". The term "nursing diagnosis" in the nursing process refers to the independent functions of the community nurse. In some literature such as Clark (1984) and Spradley (1990), nursing diagnosis is described as a separate step in the nursing process, but generally it forms part of the assessment phase.

Because of the fact that the client in community health is regarded as a total system with various kinds of needs that may influence the client's level of wellness, the nursing diagnosis will be a statement of needs rather than a list of problems. These needs will cover the whole spectrum of the health/illness continuum and can focus on a wide range of topics such as the aetiological factors or possible causes of a health problem. During this stage, priority areas as well as high-risk groups are identified. It is important to group the assessment data into specific categories and to view the classified data as a whole to make an accurate diagnosis.

After the nursing diagnosis has been made, the planning of the health care programme can begin.

2.3.2 Planning

Planning can be described as a logical, systematic, decision-making process. It requires an orderly programme of action designed around specific goals (Spradley 1990:221). Compiling a community health care plan is a complex task with multi-dimensional facets, each of which should be considered so that a comprehensive health care plan that addresses all identified needs can be provided. In community health the planning phase involves co-ordinating health care services and health care planning. This is necessary because the community nurse works with families and community groups that need and/or use multiple resources (Burgess & Ragland 1983:177).

The planning phase includes the establishment of goals and objectives, as well as the identification of intervention activities. The goal is generally a broad statement of the desired outcome, while objectives are more specific statements about the desired outcome. Intervention activities are the means by which the objectives are met. In other words, strategies that clarify what must be done to attain the objectives, the ways in which change will be initiated, and the way in which the problem cycle will be interrupted (Stanhope & Lancaster 1992:261). Objectives can be set for the long, short and intermediate terms. They must be impartial, realistic, specific and attainable within a set time.

Once again a conceptual model can be applied to facilitate the planning of the nursing action, for example Orem's self-care model, which suggests the following nursing actions: teaching, guiding, supporting and providing an environment that promotes development. Orem's self-care model provides the community nurse with the opportunity to develop an independent nursing care plan based on nursing rather than on medical needs. The nursing care plan should be able to meet all needs, and provision should be made for the promotion of health maintenance and restoration of health, as well as the prevention of illness and disability.

Planning should be a team effort in which members of the community and community leaders, as well as other health professionals, may participate to ensure that all the needs can be met and that the plan will be acceptable to the community. The plan should be put in writing and provision should be made within the plan for the expectations of all members of the team. Permanent standardised plans can be developed to meet certain general needs but should be adaptable to provide for any specific needs which are identified. All plans must be clear, easy to follow and must be regularly updated.

2.3.3 Implementation

Once the plan has been outlined, the implementation phase can begin.

Implementation can be defined as "putting the nursing care plan into action" (Ziegler *et al.* 1986:126). In other words, the community nurse must carry out the planned activities. According to Stanhope and Lancaster (1992:265), implementation is influenced "by the type of health care needs or problems, the readiness of the community to participate, the social change process, as well as the nurse's chosen role".

The first task will be to identify the knowledge and skills needed to implement the plan and decisions should be taken about the person to whom the responsibility will be delegated. The nurse usually has a leading role to play because of her knowledge and skills. She could act as a team leader, health adviser and problem-solver, and she could also distribute the work load and assign specific tasks to people with the necessary knowledge and skills. The community nurse as expert should also assist communities in the implementation of a plan, select leaders or negotiate with other experts to assist in the implementation.

Implementation requires the application of nursing theories, the establishment of a climate of trust and open communication, as well as preparing the client for accepting the planned health intervention.

During the implementation phase the independent nursing functions are the primary concern of the community nurse, but because community health intervention is a team effort, certain dependent as well as interdependent functions (such as medical treatment prescribed by a physician) will be included to meet all the needs of a client. The implementation phase is characterised by intellectual, innovative and interpersonal action and the community nurse must take the responsibility for the co-ordination of all activities. According to Yurra and Walsh (1978:120), "nurse actions are based upon a scientific rationale and directed toward promoting a suitable internal and external environment in which wellness is enhanced and illness diminished".

During the implementation phase action and reaction should be recorded because this gives direct evidence of what has been accomplished and provides guidelines for continuous problem-solving action.

During the implementation phase, selected strategies may not work, and certain changes and a reassessment of the situation will be necessary. Ongoing evaluation and openness among all members involved is essential if the implementation of selected strategies is to be facilitated.

2.3.4 Evaluation

Evaluation is usually the fourth step in the nursing process and can be described as an act of appraisal. It is an essential activity through which the effectiveness of the goal attainment can be measured. For the purposes of evaluation, standards and criteria against which the final product can be measured should be available. According to Spradley (1990:227) "the standards are the intended results of the nursing care plan, and the criteria for these standards are the specific expected client behaviours that will demonstrate the attainment of the objectives". In community nursing the purpose of the evaluation is to determine whether the planned actions meet the client needs and how well they meet these needs. It also determines whether the programme or selected strategies are relevant. The community nurse must determine the quality of care as well as the performance of the nursing personnel.

Posavac and Carey, cited by Stanhope and Lancaster (1988:211), define evaluation as "a collection of methods, skills and sensitivities necessary to determine whether a human service is needed and likely to be used, and whether it is conducted as planned, and whether the human service actually helps people in need".

There are various methods and evaluation models that can be applied to measure the outcome of community nursing care plans:

- *The structure-process-outcome model:* "Structure" refers to the evaluation of the system that provides the service, the "process" focuses on specific activities involved in the delivery of client care, while "outcome" measures the end result.
- *Formative evaluation:* This is a continuing process throughout the development of the health care plan.
- *Summative evaluation:* This deals with the outcome or end product.
- *Auditing method:* This is a review of the client's records. Retrospective auditing is the evaluation of clinical records after discharge, while current auditing is accomplished while the client is still being treated.

Evaluation is an ongoing process that starts during the assessment phase. The formative evaluation method is suitable for this purpose. The objectives formulated during the planning phase will contribute to a meaningful evaluation process. These objectives will help the nurse determine what should be evaluated. Objectives should be specific regarding the required behaviour, accomplishments and success, and must be stated from the lowest to the highest levels.

Clark (1984:213) indicates that evaluation has three facets: programme outcome, the quality of care provided and the modification required. The summative evaluation method can be applied to assess the programme outcome or the results of the programme activities. The nursing audit chart review schedule can also be used to evaluate the quality of community health care.

Proper planning for evaluation is essential and should be included in the programme planning phase. A clear, detailed outline should be given of who will be responsible, when the evaluation should take place and which methods are to be applied. It is also important to conduct a literature study on the evaluation methods and techniques used so that the most appropriate methods for a specific purpose are selected. The choice of a model or method will depend on the reasons or purpose for evaluation - whether progress, outcome or impact is to be measured.

There are various sources of information available for the evaluation of the implemented nursing activities. Consumers of health services can provide essential information regarding the acceptability of a health care service; their feelings, reactions and judgement are valuable indicators.

Evaluation is an important component in community nursing practice and the community nurse must be aware of the methods and techniques that can be applied.

2.3.5 Recording

Health records form an integral part of any health system and are an essential instrument. Health records serve as a means of communication, providing

TABLE 2.1: An example of community evaluation

Nursing diagnosis:	Increased incidence of venereal disease among teenagers in the community.
Community goal:	The community will reduce the incidence of venereal disease among teenagers by 30/07/1992.
Objective:	Appropriate community officials will develop strategies to reduce venereal disease by 30/07/1992.
Nursing orders:	*Formative evaluation*
The nurse will meet with community health department, and city council and high school personnel to discuss: (1) the increased incidence of venereal disease, (2) complications of venereal disease, and (3) venereal disease control strategies by 20/06/1990.	On 05/06/1990 the nurse and health officials met and discussed the nursing order. Three of five members expressed an interest in developing improved educational services. On 10/06/1990 the nurse and 10 members of the city health department met to discuss the nursing objectives. This department moved to increase educational services and publicity to reduce the incidence of venereal disease among teenagers. On 18/06/1990 the nurse met with six members of the high school personnel to discuss the nursing objectives. They suggested having a special programme on venereal disease.
The nurse will develop a list of strategies for improving teenagers' knowledge of the prevention and treatment of venereal disease from the suggestions made by community health members by 30/06/1990.	The nurse developed the following list of strategies from the suggestions of community members contacted above: (1) radio and television messages, (2) venereal disease pamphlets distributed in high school, (3) high school assembly on venereal disease, and (4) posters with information on signs of venereal disease and treatment clinics.
Summative evaluation Community members from the public health department, the city health department and the high school met with the nurse during June 1990 to discuss the increased incidence of venereal disease among teenagers and to suggest strategies to reduce the incidence. Each group demonstrated an interest in reducing this community concern and offered several suggestions for improving education about venereal disease and trying to reduce the incidence. Community members are aware of the problem, but the nurse will follow up and facilitate community action to improve educational service and clinic information. Some progress has been made toward goal achievement, but follow-up is necessary. More objectives are needed to achieve the goal.	

comprehensive information on the client and his or her family, the extent and quality of service rendered, any legal procedures that may have arisen (such as charges laid against nurses or other health care personnel for misconduct or negligence), training of health care personnel and research conducted.

Full, accurate and scientific documentation is of the utmost importance in any nursing service. The community nurse can by no means be absolved of this responsibility because the nature of community health care is such that

TABLE 2.2: An example of a family evaluation	
Nursing diagnosis:	Inadequate safety precautions in the home.
Family goal:	The family will eliminate safety hazards to children in their home (mutually established).
Objective 1:	The family will identify ways to remove safety hazards from their home by 05/06/1990.
Nursing orders:	*Formative evaluation*
The nurse will write a checklist of safety factors that homes with small children should have.	On 30/04/1990 the nurse, after consultation with the health department, wrote a safety checklist.
The family and nurse will discuss the checklist and the family will complete the list by 15/05/1990.	On 05/05/1990 Mr and Mrs M seemed enthusiastic on reading the checklist and agreed to fill it in during the next week.On 07/05/1990 the nurse visited the family, but they had not completed the safety list. They promised to work on it.
The family and nurse will discuss the results of the safety checklist by 20/05/1990.	On 15/05/1990 the checklist was completed and discussed with the family. Four areas were deficient and the family agreed to work on improving safety in those areas.
The family and nurse will explore ways to eliminate safety hazards in four areas by 25/05/1990.	On 20/05/1990 the family and nurse discussed several ways to remove each safety hazard.
Objective 2:	The family will remove safety hazards from their home by 30/06/1990.
The family will decide on the best way to eliminate safety hazards in their home by 01/06/1990.	The family discussed alternatives for eliminating each safety hazard and decided on a specific measure for each on 01/06/1990.
The family will implement each safety precaution they previously decided on by 21/06/1990.	On 07/06/1990 the family agreed to take the necessary measures but had not yet had time to do so. On 14/06/1990, the family showed the nurse how they had corrected each safety hazard. The family members seemed pleased by their action.
The family and nurse will evaluate the results of their safety precautions by 30/06/1990.	On 30/06/1990 the family and nurse discussed the family's feelings about precautions, and the family expressed relief and gratitude to the nurse.
Summative evaluation This family was able to identify and correct four safety hazards to their children in its home. The family took appropriate measures to eliminate safety hazards and maintained these measures. The family goal was effectively met; no further action is deemed necessary at this time.	

the client, the family, the community as well as numerous resources are involved in the programme. Documentation and record keeping are therefore necessary to ensure the effectiveness and continuity of the programme.

Documentation is an ongoing activity, starting in the assessment phase and continuing throughout all the phases. Documentation will include all information collected regarding the health history of a client, findings from physical examinations, diagnostic tests, clinical observations, treatment and the nursing care plans.

If the question of professional liability is ever raised, the recording system may be the deciding factor in the evaluation of the quality of care provided.

The problem-orientated system of record keeping is widely used in health care services and is comprised of four components, i.e. the data base, the list of problems, the nursing care plan and the progress report. The data base includes the information on solutions for the client's current problems, which should be reviewed and updated on a regular basis.

Each problem must be dealt with by care givers through action or referral.

The initial plan for each problem includes the broad goal and specific objectives that should be achieved through intervention. Progress notes are used to update the status of the problems and to document the implementation of the plan as well as the intervention results. Progress notes must be numbered, titled and dated (Clark 1984:200–201).

This system, according to Clark (1984:198), has the following advantages:

- it is directed towards total patient care;
- it is comprehensive;
- it encourages communication between members of the team;
- it is cost-effective because it eliminates duplication;
- it can be applied to quality care in measuring the effectiveness of health care programmes; and
- confidentiality is better safeguarded.

When used correctly, any member of the health care team will be able to evaluate the client's health status from the records.

Computers are increasingly utilised in health care services for storing clinical records, health histories and other data concerning the assessment, diagnosis, treatment and care of individual clients. Statistics on notifiable diseases, utilisation of services and immunisation are also computed. It is therefore essential that community nurses should be conversant with this method of record keeping.

2.4 SUMMARY

The nursing process or scientific method of nursing as a tool in the provision of community nursing is described in this chapter. The various phases of the nursing process, i.e. assessment, planning, implementation, evaluation and record keeping are outlined as they apply to community nursing.

Assessment is described as an act of appraisal of the health status and needs of the client and is regarded as the most important step of the nursing process. The nursing diagnosis is made after the collected data have been analysed and synthesised. Planning of the health care programme follows the diagnosis and this step includes the formulation of objectives and the determination of priorities and strategies. During the implementation phase the health care programme is put into action. Recording is emphasised as an important element of the nursing process because proper, comprehensive records have many advantages and can serve as a vital tool in evaluating community health care. Records also ensure continuity of health care programmes and provide comprehensive information on the client and his family.

QUESTIONS

1. Describe a method of collecting data with a view to making a nursing diagnosis in community health care.
2. Outline a community health care plan for a specific health care need in a community.

FURTHER READING

Burgess, W. & Ragland, E.C. 1983. *Community health nursing. Philosophy, process, practice.* Norwalk, Connecticut: Appleton-Century-Crofts.

Clark, M.J.D. 1996. *Community nursing. Health care for today and tomorrow.* Reston: Prentice-Hall.

Spradley, B.W. 1990. *Community nursing. Concepts and practice.* Glenview: Scott, Foresman.

BIBLIOGRAPHY

Burgess, W. & Ragland, E.C. 1983. *Community health nursing. Philosophy, process, practice.* Norwalk, Connecticut: Appleton-Century-Crofts.

Clark, M.J.D. 1984. *Community nursing. Health care for today and tomorrow.* Reston: Prentice-Hall.

Spradley, B.W. 1990. *Community health nursing. Concepts and practice.* Glenview: Scott, Foresman.

Stanhope, M. & Lancaster, J. 1988 & 1992. *Community health nursing. Process and practice for promoting health.* St Louis: Mosby.

Yurra, H. & Walsh, M.B. 1978. *The nursing process: assessing, planning, implementing, evaluating.* New York: Appleton-Century-Crofts.

Ziegler, S.M. *et al.* 1986. *Nursing process, diagnosis, nursing knowledge.* Norwalk, Connecticut: Appleton-Century-Crofts.

3 The various roles of the community nurse

MARIE DREYER

CHAPTER OBJECTIVES

After reading this chapter, the student should be able to:

- describe the advocacy role of the community nurse;
- describe the management role of the community nurse;
- describe the research role of the community nurse; and
- explain the role of the community nurse as provider of community health care.

3.1 INTRODUCTION

The community nurse is a nurse practising in the community health field, away from the formal structure of therapeutic institutions. She must be able to function independently and to take responsibility for her own actions and omissions. In South Africa she is a nurse registered under the Nursing Act, and has an additional qualification in community nursing.

Community nursing practice goes far beyond the purely physical problems of the patient. It is concerned with the prevention of disease and the promotion of health. Community nursing practice covers a wide field in the provision of health care to communities, i.e. to individuals, families and various groups. It is generally accepted that the community nurse provides an extensive, comprehensive service in various fields. She thus fulfils a variety of roles. These roles are well described in nursing literature and include roles such as those of advocate, consultant, educator, leader, caregiver and manager. Her roles and functions are controlled by rules and regulations for nursing practice, health legislation and other applicable legislation and policies.

A role can be described as the expected or assumed performance assigned to a person in a given situation or position. Each role implies certain functions, tasks and responsibilities. The term "role" is generally defined as "the functioning of individuals in a group and the learning of a social role as an aspect of personality that is acquired with other habits" (Edelman & Mandle 1990:12). The role of the community nurse refers to the expected functions and performance of a specific category of nurse. The norms, standards, functions and codes of conduct are determined by a statutory body such as the Nursing Council. According to Clark (1984:44), "the specific role of the community nurse is in continual transition, responding to the changing needs of the community she serves". She also maintains that not every community nurse will engage in all the role functions identified.

3.2 THE ROLE OF THE COMMUNITY NURSE AS AN ADVOCATE

The most fundamental principle in any nursing process is that of the nurse's role as advocate, as it is based on the general humanitarian principle of recognition of the value of humanity and on an acceptance of the unique relationship between the nurse and the consumer of health care. The patient as a human being is the central focus and the individual is regarded as a unique being with his or her own physical, psychological, intellectual, spiritual and social characteristics and needs that have to be taken into consideration at all times.

Advocacy in community health care should not be confused with the legal connotation of the word "advocate", i.e. one who defends his client. Advocacy, in the context of community health care delivery, is both an action in support of the consumer of health care services and a provision of information to that consumer. In her role as advocate, the community nurse's aim is to support her client and to provide him with advice and information. The individual's independence and his sense of human dignity and personal freedom are impeded and adversely affected by illness. It is thus the task of the nurse to meet the individual's needs during this time of crisis and to support and assist the client until he or she is able to resume a normal life. Spradley and Allender (1996:665) define the advocacy role of the community nurse as:

> a role in which the nurse acts or speaks on behalf of clients to help clients to gain greater independence or self-determination and to make the system more responsive and relevant to their needs.

The essence of this humanitarian intervention and aid is the development of a dynamic interpersonal relationship between nurse and client. This is primarily a visible expression of the empathy and sense of dignity that an individual has with regard to him- or herself and others. For some people, a humanitarian act is part of their daily life-styles, while for others it is the result of deliberate effort. It can thus be said that the nurse's role as advocate is based on humanitarianism and on an inner compulsion to render assistance.

The basis of formal assistance lies in the assumption that the community nurse has at her disposal the necessary knowledge, ability and skill to provide her client with support and advice. She intervenes when the individual, family or community is no longer in a position to deal with a health problem or crisis. The goals of her intervention are defined in conjunction with her patient, and the necessary referrals are made when the nurse does not have the appropriate knowledge or skill to take action herself. The entire process of advocacy lies primarily in the conduct of the nurse and in the unique situation of the client. Actions are strongly influenced by good communication and mutual respect, and the manner in which the particular needs and circumstances of the client are defined.

According to Stanhope and Lancaster (1992:682), the functions of advocacy require "scientific knowledge, expert communication, facilitation skills, and problem-solving and affirmation techniques". The goal of advocacy must always be to promote self-determination and independence. Continued informed permission and decision-making for action are essential, and expectations and responsibilities must be respected to ensure the success of co-operation. Each individual's particular needs, values and beliefs must be taken into account and the client's rights must remain the focus of priority. Information provided should always be correct and on such a level that the client will be able to understand it.

The community nurse must be attuned to delivering a compassionate service and thus support the individual as a whole. The client must be helped in such a way that he or she is able to attain independence and to take responsibility for his or her own life and health. Health workers should be cautioned against taking the client's decisions on his or her behalf. As a result of their knowledge of illness and health, nurses tend to dominate their patients and clients and to take decisions for them rather than to work together with them.

In addition, the advocacy role is also directed towards dealing with those authorities and organisations involved with health and health care delivery and to enter into discussions and negotiations with them to ensure that the consumer's needs can be met. The consumer's needs should thus be pin-pointed through surveys and opinion polls. The community nurse's primary task is to provide the consumer with health care services that are readily available, accessible and affordable (Spradley 1990) and it may therefore sometimes be necessary to collect data and to present the findings to encourage funding, for example for shelter for the homeless.

The nurse's role as advocate may include a variety of functions that could be influenced by the client's needs and environment. These functions may vary from the promotion of her client's interests to acting as mediator and facilitator for decision making as well as to negotiating for services for poor people, children, refugees, etc. In a complex and sometimes fragmented health care delivery system the clients often need someone to explain which services they ought to use. This is particularly true for the poor and for minorities. Spradley and Allender (1996:106) maintain that "whether the population is homeless people, battered women, migrant workers or some other group the community nurse in the advocate role speaks or acts on their behalf". The most essential characteristics required of the nurse in her role as advocate are the following:

- a good understanding of human rights;
- a willingness to take a chance;
- an ability to communicate and to be persuasive;
- an ability to negotiate and to identify resources; and
- an ability to co-ordinate and to co-operate.

3.3 THE MANAGEMENT ROLE OF THE COMMUNITY NURSE

The community nurse, like all other categories of nurses, is responsible for the management of client services. Her management function involves supervising family health care, running clinics, planning health care programmes, referring clients to other health care professionals, etc. It is particularly in the community health care field that the community nurse co-ordinates and integrates all the facilities and resources available so that a comprehensive health care service, which meets all health care needs in a specific community, can be provided. Management can in this regard be described as "the administrative process of mobilising, deploying, supervising, and evaluating human and other resources to achieve the health care objectives" (WHO 1979:411).

The management role of the community nurse includes the systematic co-ordination of activities, objectives, strategies and application of policies to meet the organisational goal, for example the provision of a comprehensive health care service. The management role also comprises planning, organisation, leadership and evaluation functions. The community nurse as manager of community health care delivery must aim at high productivity and encourage all members of her staff to provide quality health care services. She must be sufficiently competent to organise her services in such a way that the clients and personnel of the organisation for which she works will be satisfied. Community nurse managers should show sensitivity to external political, social, economic and physical influences (WHO 1979:412).

The community nurse must have a sound philosophy and a knowledge of the values and traditions of the community to be served. Within the parameters of the policy of the organisation, her scope of practice, the applicable legislation and the needs of the community, she must plan, organise and evaluate the community nursing services. Her management role will vary according to the complexity, mission and objectives of the organisation.

Lock (1989:30–34) emphasises the following elements from Mintzberg's model of management roles:

- *The interpersonal role:* This specifies the role of the nurse/manager as symbolic head, leader and liaison officer.

- *The informational role:* This is concerned with receiving, transmitting and distributing information to members of the organisation as well as to people outside.
- *The decision-making role:* This covers facets of conflict and grievance management, negotiation, allocation of resources and supervision of projects. Decision-making forms an integral part of all management functions and the community nurse as manager must have specific skills and knowledge to make the right decisions and to resolve problems in various situations.

The community nurse must be aware of both the formal and informal structures within the organisation as well as the lines of authority and communication within and between these structures. She should be able to negotiate with leaders in the community as well as with health authorities to provide the necessary resources and facilities for the development of a comprehensive health care service. In providing health care in the community health field, she has to co-operate and liaise with the various members of the health team, organisations and members of the community.

As allocator of resources, the community nurse manager is responsible for ensuring that adequate supplies, equipment, drugs, material, communication systems, transport and manpower are readily available. According to the World Health Organisation (1979), managers must be continually aware of the quality and quantity of available resources, and must also be capable of making the required adjustments. An adequate, continuous flow of resources to community health care services is a fundamental requirement. Lock (1989:34) indicates that to be able to promote efficiency, economy and productivity, standardised norms must be established for storage, distribution, supervision and control of resources.

One of the most important management functions of the community nurse is supervision. The constant supervision of health care delivery provided by the community health personnel, such as immunisation, home health care or health education services, is essential to ensure that quality health care services are provided. As supervisor she will have to delegate responsibility to her subordinates within the health care service. Delegated responsibility should be accompanied by the necessary authority as well as accountability, but the supervisor remains responsible for the performance of her subordinates and for any neglect of their duties. In rural areas this can become a dilemma for the community nurse who is responsible for the supervision of a large area. She may be unable to visit all sections each day and this could be particularly problematic where there is a shortage of reliable senior personnel (Hein & Nicholson 1986:366).

In the community health field the nurse manager also has an advocacy duty. She is committed to support the health personnel to resolve problems regarding grievances and frustrations. In rural areas lack of reliable transport and communication systems, unattractive working and living conditions, as well as delayed payment of salaries are often sources of great frustration, and here particularly the community nurse manager must be competent and able to support her staff. She will have to negotiate with the people concerned to solve the problems and to improve the conditions. She may also have to counsel health personnel on their personal problems and conflicts.

3.3.1 The role of the community nurse manager as a leader

One of the major functions of the community nurse is that of leader. She directs the implementation of the health care plan and develops new approaches to solving problems. As leader of the health care team, she acts as coordinator, teacher and evaluator of the team efforts. She uses leadership skills to create an environment that allows for the development of skills and strategies for the improvement of health care.

According to Stanhope and Lancaster (1992:654), "leaders tend to view work as an enabling process, involving some combination of people and ideas interacting to establish strategies and make decisions". As leader, the community nurse serves as a role model for all people with whom she comes into contact, such as clients, student nurses and other professionals. The leadership role of the community nurse involves guiding, decision-making, stimulating interest in health promotion, directing disease prevention programmes, initiating therapy and influencing health-related policies. The community nurse manager should therefore be knowledgeable and assertive if she is to act as a leader who is able to persuade other professionals, as well as health authorities, to provide the necessary health care services that will satisfy the community's health care needs.

The community nurse manager as a leader also has a vital role to play in the attainment of the goal of health for all by the year 2000. She must have a clear understanding of the strategies involved and the implementation thereof. She must develop a deep understanding of the philosophy of primary health care and be able to mobilise communities to participate in reaching the goal.

3.3.2 The role of the community nurse manager as evaluator of community health care

Evaluation is a continuous process aimed at correcting and improving a situation or a procedure carried out repeatedly. Feedback techniques provide the information needed for the adjustment and the setting of performance objectives. This facilitates the evaluation task of community health care managers.

In the final analysis, the community nurse manager should evaluate all the actions implemented (such as nursing care, health care programmes and staff performances). She is also responsible for planning evaluation programmes and managing the evaluation process. Management of the evaluation process requires decisions to be made about the most suitable methods or models for a specific programme, the evaluation that should take place, who should be involved, and which methods for the analysis of data would be the most appropriate.

Ongoing evaluation is essential, as it is through this process that it can be determined whether reorganisation is needed. During the evaluation process the community nurse manager must re-examine the original plan, the utilisation of human and material resources and the degree to which all objectives are being attained. It should be remembered that the community nurse is responsible and accountable to both the employer and the profession. It is essential, therefore, that the community nurse as manager must be aware of the standards and criteria established for quality community health care and that in this regard she should realise her responsibility in ensuring that high standards are achieved. Only if she ensures this will she be able to prevent legal action being taken against her, the organisation or the personnel under her supervision.

High standards can be maintained through regular inspection, supervision and evaluation of the services rendered. The community nurse must improve her management skills through continuing education and regularly update her knowledge.

The application of the management process by the community nurse is essential. She must be able to co-ordinate and supervise the efforts of her subordinates to reach the goals determined by the health care organisation.

A knowledge of more recent developments and techniques, such as the computerisation of records and classification systems, contributes to a more streamlined management process. The management role of the community nurse is challenging and can be very rewarding when the goal is achieved. Effective management is a key factor in the optimal utilisation of the available resources (WHO 1979). According to Lock (1989:207), "the management roles are seen as central to the administrative process within the nursing service and central to the integration of these services within the domains of a complex comprehensive health system".

3.4 THE EDUCATIONAL ROLE OF THE COMMUNITY NURSE

The community nurse has an important role to play as educator to both health personnel and consumers of health care. The educational role comprises, among others, health education, in-service training, orientation and formal teaching and training. The community nurse must be able to plan, co-ordinate and manage the various educational programmes in the health care service. She must determine the specific learning needs of the community, students and other health care workers. She must also ensure that the teaching and training programmes are relevant for the specific target group, country or population.

Clark (1984:47) claims that community nurses spend ninety per cent of their time in some educational activity. This may involve formal lectures to groups, informal sharing of information with a client, or demonstrating a baby bath to a new mother.

3.4.1 In-service education

This function is an essential element of the teaching role of the community nurse. In-service education is that given to a person while he or she is employed to do a specific job. Mellish (1978:11) defines in-service education as follows:

> It is part of continuing education but not the whole of it. It is deliberately planned education to meet the needs of a specific employer, by making up deficiencies in technical and scientific information in his employees.

The community nurse is responsible for determining the specific deficiencies in the knowledge or skills of the community health personnel and for planning the necessary programmes according to these needs. Regular in-service education for personnel is necessary to keep them abreast of new developments and technology. It is also a valuable instrument in promoting the delivery of quality community health care. Because nurses working in the community health field (especially in rural areas in South Africa) are isolated and often have to work on their own, in-service education is of great importance, as it keeps them up to date on new developments, health policies, legislation and treatment regimes.

3.4.2 Orientation

Orientation is the introduction of new personnel to the environment or to the relevant policies, procedures, philosophies, purpose and personnel benefits of the organisation where they are employed. It is the responsibility of the community nurse to plan and implement such a programme of orientation for all newly-appointed staff. Regular evaluation and updating of the programme is essential. Aspects such as the storage of vaccines to retain the cold chain in rural areas, the organisation and provision of primary health care through mobile units, storage of medication, dealing with emergencies, etc. can be covered in these programmes. The importance of orientation lies in the fact that the newly appointed community nurse will know what is expected of her and that she will be up to date regarding her scope of practice.

3.4.3 Health education

This is one of the most important elements of the community nurse's educational role. It forms an integral part of the daily functions of the community nurse and, according to the World Health Organisation (1988), the objectives are to enable people:

- to define their own problems and needs;
- to understand what they can do about these problems with their own resources combined with outside support; and
- to decide on the most appropriate action to promote healthy living and community well-being.

Health education is a process that prepares people for making health-related decisions such as to stop smoking or to use health resources. In health education, the emphasis is on changes in health behaviour. The role and functions of the community nurse are to plan, implement, co-ordinate, supervise and evaluate both the programmes as well as the outcome of any health education presented. She must conduct research so that she can determine whether health behaviour has changed, or whether the needs and problems of specific target groups have changed. A thorough knowledge of learning and teaching principles is necessary to make a success of health education. The contents of the health education programme vary according to the situation and particular needs encountered. Clark (1984:47) indicates that the most effective educational tool is the community nurse herself, as she serves as a role model for her clients.

Health education is an instrument for the prevention of disease and the promotion of health. It forms the foundation of primary health care and is an important method of transmitting messages about the modification of life-styles and/or health behaviour, as well as about prevention of diseases, to as many people as possible. The community nurse has an important role to play in this regard because of the time she spends in direct contact with her clients, which in turn provides ample opportunity for disseminating knowledge.

3.4.4 Teaching of community health care personnel

Apart from her role as health educator, the community nurse is also responsible for the teaching and training of student nurses, primary health care workers and other categories of health personnel, such as traditional healers and midwives. She must plan programmes for student nurses for their clinical experience in the community health field, and act as supervisor and evaluator for these students. She has a major responsibility to train primary health care workers and to guide and supervise them in case-finding, disease prevention, patient and family care, community development as well as in presenting health education. The community nurse is also responsible for developing relevant educational models or programmes for primary health care workers. Training programmes should also be organised for supervisors, teachers of primary health care workers and other categories of health personnel. Short courses can be planned and offered to satisfy specifically the learning needs of community nurses practising in rural areas in the community.

Teaching is inherent in the nurse's role and she teaches patients, families, ancillary personnel and other nurses (Spradley 1990). Her knowledge and competence in this regard must be continually updated.

3.5 THE RESEARCH ROLE OF THE COMMUNITY NURSE

The community nurse also has a research function, which may be carried out at several levels in the community health field. Spradley (1990:200) states that "research in community health, from the simplest inquiry to the most complex epidemiologic study, uses the same fundamental process". In other words, all the steps of the research process are followed, i.e. identifying an area of interest, specifying the problem, reviewing the literature, conceptualising and selecting the research design, collecting and analysing data, and interpreting the results.

The community nurse has an important role to play in conducting research. Participating in epidemiological as well as other research is essential in community health care delivery. Epidemiological data provide the community health care personnel with valuable information about specific diseases or nursing care problems on which the planning for intervention can be based.

The community nurse can undertake and plan an individual research project; conversely she may become a member of a research team. She can contribute towards the systematic identification and analysis of diseases, their aetiology, causes and distribution. She may be required to make field observations. For example, she may study the secondary attack rate within a small community, such as a family or classroom.

Research on aspects of community nursing is complex, as it is concerned with people and community factors that are continually changing. The scope of nursing research in the community health field can include all the facets of community nursing science such as the rehabilitative, therapeutic, preventative and promotive aspects of community health care delivery, education and administration.

Clark (1984:488) indicates that community nurses should know enough of the principles of research to recognise areas suitable for research and to carry out research independently. Research to strengthen the prevention of communicable disease and to improve the quality of life in developing areas is, according to the World Health Organisation (1983), of great importance and the community nurse can play an important role in this regard. She must search for new ways to control environmental hazards and to improve the health of the community.

Community nurses carry out research at many levels and this research forms an integral part of community nursing practice. This helps to determine specific needs, to evaluate the effectiveness of care and to develop theoretical bases for community health practice (Spradley 1990:202).

3.6 THE ROLE OF THE COMMUNITY NURSE AS PROVIDER OF COMMUNITY HEALTH CARE

The role of the community nurse practitioner covers a wide field and is comprehensive in nature. Her role is to serve the community as a whole and to provide for all the health care needs. In the South African context the community nurse is involved in the provision of a comprehensive health care service. The scope of her practice is regulated by the legislation and rules of nursing practice, health legislation and other relevant acts of the country.

Within the comprehensive health care system, the community nurse fulfils the roles and functions related to the prevention of disease, the promotion of health and the provision of curative and rehabilitative health care.

The community nurse is also responsible for providing health care at primary, secondary and tertiary levels to all age groups, from before birth until death, in clinics, health care centres, at home or through mobile units in rural areas. Because of the high cost of hospitalisation, patients are discharged at an early stage and cared for in the home setting. The community nurse has a role to play in discharge planning and the follow-up care of these patients. Community nurses are also, to an increasing extent, involved in the care of patients on support systems in the home. This requires high technical and clinical skills, knowledge and competence. The role and functions of the community nurse in the management of high-technology health care in the home setting includes the co-ordination of team members and the planning and delivery of health care. She co-ordinates the visits of the various team members, arranges emergency visits and is also responsible for the control and maintenance of supplies as well as the equipment. In addition, she is responsible for obtaining laboratory specimens and keeping the family and team members informed (Cookfair 1991:385).

One of the most important functions of the community nurse is, according to Clark (1984:46), the assessment of the client's needs, planning interventions to meet these needs, and implementing and evaluating the plan. To an increasing extent community nurses are required to become involved in the diagnosis and treatment of patients and clients in the community health care setting. In South Africa special legislation was promulgated to enable community nurses to carry out these functions under certain circumstances. The specific legislation promulgated is associated with the Nursing Amendment Act 71 of 1981, Section 38A of the Nursing Act, as amended, as well as the Amendment Act of 1982. According to the new health plan for South Africa, community nurses will play an important role in providing primary health care and great emphasis is placed on their clinical competence.

Health care roles of the community nurse relate to services such as school health, occupational health, mother and child care, community mental health, health education and care for the aged in urban as well as rural areas.

The growing urban population of South Africa, with squatter camps on the peripheries of the cities, also places an additional responsibility on community nurses, as disease prevention and the promotion of health of the people in these settlements is extremely important. This task is difficult, as primary health care services are often provided in these areas under dangerous and difficult circumstances.

The community nurse is also responsible for environmental health and must be aware and well informed about possible environmental health hazards. She should constantly assess aspects such as water and air pollution, infectious agents, safety issues and other stresses that may affect the health status of the population. She must report on these to the appropriate health authorities and negotiate with managers of factories, etc. to use more environment-friendly methods and products to prevent pollution. She should also urge industries to take the necessary precaution to prevent the spillage of toxic agents in the environment, which could pollute food or water resources.

3.7 SUMMARY

The dynamics of health care and disease require constant updating of the knowledge and skills of community nurses. New diseases such as AIDS must be dealt with and the community nurse should have some knowledge regarding the prevention and treatment of these diseases as well as an awareness of the ethical issues that she may encounter in this regard.

The community nurse will play an increasingly important role in the future health care provision in South Africa, especially as the shift from expensive curative health care to community-based health care delivery, with its emphasis on the prevention of disease and the promotion of health, becomes a reality. Her role in these services is therefore considered vital to the optimum development of these services. This presents the community nurse with enormous challenges and responsibilities.

QUESTIONS

1. Outline the management role of the community nurse in a school health service.
2. Discuss the supervising role of the community nurse.
3. Describe the role of the community nurse as provider of community health care.

FURTHER READING

Clark, M.J.D. 1996. *Community health care for today and tomorrow*. Relevant chapters. Reston: Prentice-Hall

Spradley, B.W. 1990. *Community health nursing. Concepts and practice.* Relevant chapters. Glenview: Scott, Foresman.

Stanhope, M. & Lancaster, J. 1992. *Community health nursing. Process and practice for promoting health.* Part 7. St Louis: Mosby.

BIBLIOGRAPHY

Clark, M.J.D. 1984. *Community health care for today and tomorrow.* Reston: Prentice-Hall.

Cookfair, J.M. 1991. *Nursing process and practice in the community.* St Louis: Mosby.

Edelman, C.L. & Mandle, C.L. 1990. *Health promotion throughout the lifespan.* St Louis: Mosby.

Hein, E.C. & Nicholson, M.J. 1986. *Contemporary leadership behavior: selected readings.* Boston: Little, Brown and Company.

Lock, M.V.L.H. 1989. "The role of the nurse administrator in rural hospitals in the Republic of South Africa". Unpublished doctoral thesis.

Mellish, J.M. 1978. *Theory and methods of in-service education for nurses.* Pretoria: South African Nursing Association.

Spradley, B.W. 1990. *Community health nursing. Concepts and practice.* Glenview: Scott, Foresman.

Spradley, B.W. & Allender, J.A. 1996. *Community health nursing. Concepts and practice.* Philadelphia: Lippencott.

Stanhope, M. & Lancaster, J. 1992. *Community health nursing. Process and practice for promoting health.* St Louis: Mosby.

WHO. 1979. "Development of rural health teams. Views of a WHO expert committee." *WHO Chronicle,* 33:403–14.

WHO. 1983. "World health day 1983. Health for all: the countdown has begun." *WHO Chronicle,* 37(2):65–70.

WHO. 1988. *Education for health. A manual on health education in primary health care.* Geneva: World Health Organisation.

4 Demography

SUSAN HATTINGH

CHAPTER OBJECTIVES

After reading this chapter, the student should be able to:

- explain the concepts of demography and population;
- put into perspective the global problems that uncontrolled population growth may cause;
- put into perspective how the nurse may contribute to the handling of the problems that uncontrolled population growth may cause; and
- describe the importance of the knowledge of demography with regard to health care and planning.

4.1 INTRODUCTION

The science of demography has a long history of attempts to describe population phenomena in terms of one universal population contingency. Today this science has developed to such an extent that we can, to a certain extent, predict the future of mankind. The era in which we live is marked by the most dramatic population changes in human existence and even with sophisticated scientific predictions made by demographers and other scientists, the destiny of the human race cannot be predicted with certainty.

There is a definite complex interaction between the demographic characteristics of a population, its health status and its health needs. In this chapter an outline will be given of the factors that influence the size and composition of populations, the present status of the world population and, in particular, the South African situation, and the current trends in the South African population.

The community nurse has an important task in the destiny of the population, as her role is seen as a key to the development and health of the population.

With this chapter an attempt is made to present a brief demographic profile of the South African population. The information included here is that which is currently available. The objective is to give the community nurse a broad background on the influence of population changes, for example the influence of population growth on health, the environment and the social structure of the community.

Population and the environment go hand in hand. Both affect the practice of nurses because they are the people who serve the community in all its facets. With the emphasis on primary health care, nurses may no longer ignore the effect of demographic factors on the epidemiology of the population. A knowledge of the total community and the environment in which it lives, works, plays and multiplies is essential for a study of disease profiles. Nurses are equal partners in the delivery of health care, thus their knowledge will determine the value of their contribution.

4.2 THE HISTORIC DEVELOPMENT OF DEMOGRAPHY

The history of demography can be traced back to Biblical times when population registration systems were instated. Although this census system is now somewhat more sophisticated, it is still being used to determine the characteristics of the population.

The current population explosion is relatively recent. Until 1750 the world population was no more than 791 million and its size was stable. There was a high fertility rate, but also an equally high mortality rate, which fluctuated from year to year, depending on natural disasters, floods, droughts and plagues. Even in times of prosperity, death rates were high, thus preventing soaring population growth.

It was only in about 1750 that these patterns started to change and between 1750 and about 1900, the world population figure increased five times.

The much criticised English priest, historian and amateur student of mathematics and economics, Thomas R. Malthus (1766–1834), wrote his renowned *Essay on the Principle of Population, or a View of its Past and Present Effects on Human Happiness, with an Inquiry into Our Prospects Respecting the Future Removal or Mitigation of the Evils Which It Occasions* in 1798. Malthus described the interrelationship between population numbers and the available means of sustaining life. He stated that if the population could not contain itself by means of moral control, a celibate life-style and prolonging of marriages, then the available resources would decrease to such an extent that there would be social deviations, immorality, epidemics, diseases and hunger.

Malthus pointed out that human populations increase geometrically (that is, by multiplication – 2,4,8,16,32), while the food supply increases arithmetically (by addition – 2,4,6,8). He believed that food supply served as a check on human populations. If there were to be a decline in the population as a result of war, starvation and diseases, this would enable food production to catch up, and the process of growth and eventual decline would start all over.

Malthus's theory predicted that no uplifting of standards or increase in productivity could control the events that were seen as an inescapable vicious circle – the human race was doomed to failure. Malthus also realised that very few people would voluntarily abstain from sexual relations or be celibate and he therefore saw this very grim future of the human race as inevitable.

Malthus's theory did not foresee the increase in the standard of living in developed countries, birth control measures and production of food through highly sophisticated technology, nor did he predict the attendant decline in population growth, but his ghost still looms in developing countries and many scientists believe that his theory is correct after all.

Although the work and predictions of Malthus were much criticised, he stimulated others such as William Farr (who was the first to develop the British census) and the leaders in the field of birth control. Their studies led to the realisation that a knowledge of the population is vitally important for the administrative, political, economic and academic fields.

It was only after World War I that more scientists started realising the importance of vital processes and it was A.M. Carr-Saunders's publication, *The Population Problem: a study in Evolution* written in 1922, that resulted in an interest in and recognition of population science at an international level (Raubenheimer 1987:2).

FIGURE 4.1: The Malthusian theory of population growth versus food supply

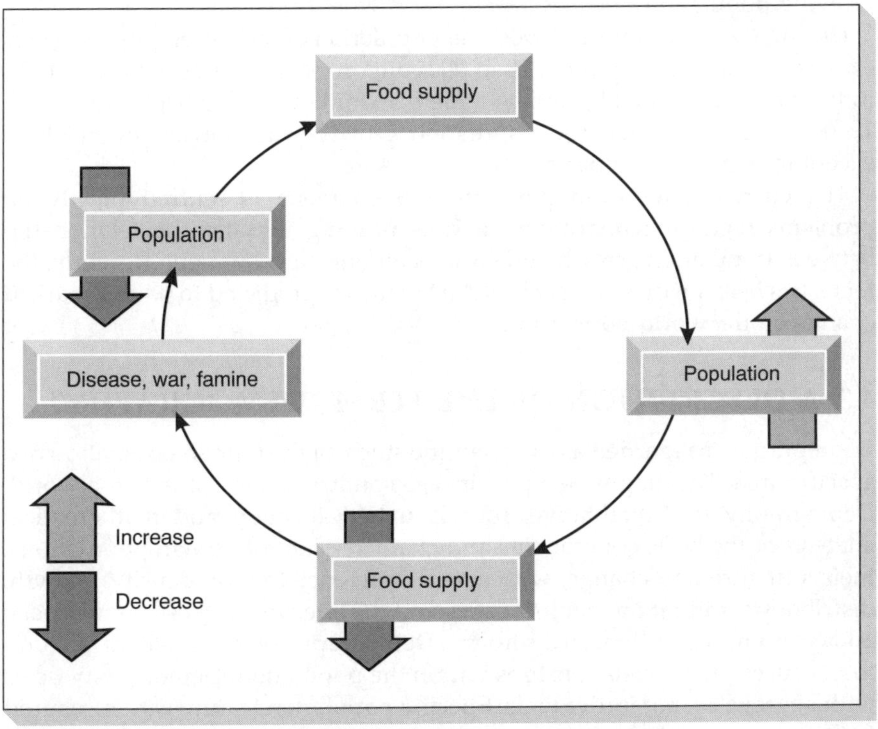

It was during the twentieth century, with all its advances in medical technology and the introduction of sanitary and health-related measures, that a marked growth rate occurred. It was, however, during the 1970s that a slackening of the growth rate was noted, but only in developed countries. In developing countries, which are also the poorest countries of the world, a soaring population growth was recorded.

It was as a result of concern about uncontrolled population growth and the possibility of a threat to the population of the world, that the first international congress on demography was held in Geneva in 1972. This was followed by the establishment of the International Union for the Scientific Study of Population Problems. After this, the International Institute of Statistics was established, where international demographic information was collected.

It was noted with concern that the world population was growing at an average rate of 1,7 per cent per annum. By the turn of the century, the current world population of 5,4 billion people would have increased to 6,2 billion. The momentum of population growth resulted in the addition of at least another 3 billion people between 1985 and 2025. Over 90% of the growth is taking place in the developing world; these developing countries are least able to cope with the resources and environmental consequences of the growing population.

During the course of the 1990s, the population of the developing world is expected to increase by more than 900 million, while the population of the industrial countries will grow by a mere 56 million. At the beginning of the 1980s, it appeared that the population growth was slowing everywhere except in Africa and in parts of Southern Asia.

The current interest in population phenomena is centred mostly on problems regarding migration, urbanisation, ageing and the relationship between population growth and socio-economic development. Recently, the focus has been on diseases such as AIDS that are predicted to have a marked change on the world population.

4.3 A DESCRIPTION OF THE TERM "DEMOGRAPHY"

Demography is regarded as the scientific study of the human population of a specific area. This might be a province, a country, a continent or the world. Demography is a qualitative, formal statistical study and mathematical analysis of the basic components and characteristics of human populations, their structure and change, with special reference to size, density, growth, distribution, migration, vital statistics and the effect of all these on the social and economic conditions in a country. Demography is thus a scientific study that focuses on interrelationships within the population. Demography deals with aggregates, not individuals. Specific population features are measured for a total population or segments of it and compared to similar figures for previous years or other countries. Demography is therefore easily presented in tables and graphs because it is fundamentally descriptive and analytical rather than explanatory.

4.4 A DESCRIPTION OF THE TERM "POPULATION"

The term "population" refers to a group of people resident within a specific geographical area, who are identified by one or more common characteristics such as their place of residence. Alternatively, these characteristics could be racial, political, religious and/or cultural. A specific population may be identified by its size, distribution or composition:

- *Size:* The size of a population is the number of individuals in a given territory at a given time. The size of a territorial population is affected by births, deaths and migration.
- *Distribution:* The distribution of a population is the spatial arrangement of individuals within the given territory at a given time, for example rural and urban distribution. This distribution indicates the density of the population.
- *Composition:* The composition of a population is the assortment of individual characteristics within the population, such as age, sex, race and marital status, occupation, education, religion and language.

4.5 SOURCES OF DEMOGRAPHIC DATA

Demographic data are obtained through censuses, vital statistics (such as deaths, births and marriages) and periodical sample surveys. The last census in South Africa took place in the early 1990s but was carried out during a time of marked civil unrest, negative publication, political turmoil and disagreements. Thus the data cannot claim to be comprehensive and are at best merely estimates, especially among the black population.

There are four principal sources of recent demographic information in South Africa:

- The national census, which was conducted in 1991.
- A series of demographic surveys conducted by the Human Sciences Research Council (HSRC) from 1987 to 1989 for the Department of National Health and Population Development. The methodology used and the quality of the data obtained are debatable and the reliability is often questioned. The results, however, are being extensively used by researchers and policy makers.
- Monthly surveys were conducted until 1991 by the Central Statistical Services (CSS) to monitor the short-term changes in the labour market forces. These monthly surveys included information on basic demographic changes and characteristics. An annual household survey has replaced the monthly survey since 1993. The results are widely circulated to interested parties. These surveys are viewed as extremely important, especially by policy makers, as they reflect the standard of living of the population.
- A project for statistics on living standards and development has been initiated by the University of Cape Town. This project was sponsored by the World Bank in 1993.

In addition, various official, academic and other departments and institutions, particularly researchers of the University of South Africa, The Development Bank of Southern Africa, the University of Stellenbosch, etc., have produced secondary data on censuses and related official statistics.

4.5.1 The characteristics of a census

A census is the largest single data collection exercise carried out in a country. Its characteristics are as follows:

- a complete record is made of the entire population within a geographically precisely defined area at a given time;
- each person is enumerated separately; and
- a census has a legal basis, making it compulsory to be included and to provide the information requested.

In countries where there are many illiterate people, an enumerator (a person employed to conduct the census) completes the forms, which contain a few simple, factual questions.

Census questions are short, partly because of the increasing unwillingness of individuals to fill in long forms with complex questions as well as the time, cost and effort involved in reproducing the information in a statistical format with a minimum of errors.

4.5.2 A sample survey

The most common feature of a survey is that it involves only a sample of a population. The advantage of sampling is that it reduces the effort, cost and manpower required in comparison with a census. The possibility of the introduction of a sampling error is, however, greater.

Surveys are important sources of demographic data because they eliminate the problems experienced in census taking, for example the impossibility of asking many or complex questions and, especially in developing countries, the poor quality and unmotivated response they produce.

They are relative cheap, are processed quickly and can gather much more detail than a census, including additional information. The interviewers can be much more intensively trained.

4.5.3 Vital registration

In almost all developed countries, vital registrations provide a main source of information on births, deaths, marriages and migration. The systems are often seriously incomplete and are sometimes not even used for demographic purposes.

4.6 THE LIMITATIONS OF DEMOGRAPHY

Demographic data in most countries, especially in developing countries, provide only a rough approximation of the size, distribution and sex composition of a population. It is estimated that at least 30 per cent (in some developing countries up to 50 per cent) of the world's population is not accounted for in demographic data collected through censuses.

Censuses also fail to enumerate a sizeable portion of the population. In addition, they may count many people twice and are often unreliable when it comes to distinguishing between single, married, divorced and separated persons.

Comparisons between countries are often extremely difficult and major adjustments must be made before any population data can be compared.

Reliable statistics on mortality, especially on infant mortality, are frequently unavailable and records on births, marriages, divorces and deaths are usually not kept up to date.

There are still many populations throughout the world of which we know nothing and which are not accounted for in the available data.

In South Africa, one of the mayor weaknesses of the data collected before 1993 was the exclusion of the former homelands (Transkei, Bophuthatswana, Venda, Ciskei). These former homelands accounted for a substantial proportion of the South African population. The problem of having separate governments in each homeland exacerbated the problem.

The dramatic changes that have taken place since 1993 have had profound implications for this country and data have yet to be collected to indicate the full impact.

Although it may seem that demographic data are not absolutely correct, one must not underestimate their usefulness in both planning and research.

A national census is planned for 1996 and only if these data can be proven to be representative and reliable, will the task of reconstruction, representation and detailed explanation of the South African population be viewed and regarded with a high level of scientific confidence. The nurse has a vital role to play in the census. She is an essential figure in the collection of data and the recording of vital events. Her role must never be underestimated, but may only be fully realised if she has the knowledge, expertise, ability and insight to see the importance of accurately collected data. To collect precise, reliable and truthful objective data should be a life-long policy and second nature to all nurses, irrespective of where they work.

4.7 THE PHASES OF DEMOGRAPHIC TRANSITION

Demographic transition is the term used to describe the process by which pre-industrialised populations with a high mortality and fertility rate are transformed into modern populations with a low fertility and mortality rate. There are three different phases of this transition process:

- The first phase is described as the demographic trend over a specific period marked by stability in age and sex composition or the stability of a high death and birth rate. During this phase, biological survival is threatened by any new epidemic that may reduce the population and cause an imbalance. The population is therefore vulnerable to any sudden change, be it natural disasters, man-made disasters (for example, war) or disease. Some developing countries are still in this phase of demographic transition, as there are insufficient means for providing for the health care needs of the population. Poor living standards and low production levels are the most obvious features of this phase.

- The second demographic transition phase is marked by a reduction in the death rate without a corresponding decline in the birth rate. This is a typical trend found in developing countries and is known to demographers as the "demographic gap". This rapid increase in the population may lead to considerable health and social problems, and is associated with a struggle for power. In this phase there is an imbalance between food production and other resources that are vital for sustaining life, as well as a disparity between the availability of services and the demand for these services by the rapidly growing population. Poverty, rural-urban migration, social instability and pressure on the available land suitable for agriculture and food production may result in numerous health problems.
- Phase three of the demographic transition is seen in developed countries, where the demographic gap is closed by a decreasing birth rate and higher life expectancy. This results in a more stable demographic picture. The standard of living and the general socio-economic conditions of the people in this population are much higher than in the other two phases. Health-related problems differ because there is an ageing population, which in itself is not a health problem but is associated with chronic diseases that lead to long-term treatment and care. Thus the increasing number of older people who are disabled is a major health hazard in this particular demographic phase.

4.8 THE COMPONENTS OF POPULATION GROWTH

There are basically three components that determine the population in an area. They are births (fertility), deaths (mortality) and migration. These seemingly uncomplicated phenomena can have very complex causes and results, which may considerably influence health care delivery. Behind these three components is a myriad complex social forces that the community nurse must understand, as they will determine the course of the country in which we live. Nurses will want answers to questions such as:

- Will the population continue to grow at its present rate?
- For how long?
- How will this population growth affect the health status in the country?
- What are the prospects for the future?

The balance between these factors will determine whether the population decreases, increases or remains stable. The relationship between births and deaths is referred to as the natural increase or decrease of a population. When the net effect of migration is added, the result is referred to as the total increase or decrease in a population.

4.8.1 Fertility

There are many factors that influence the fertility of individuals and communities as a whole, such as religious beliefs, cultural perspectives and views, people's average age at marriage and the population's sex ratio (the proportion of males to females). It is now widely accepted that fertility should be controlled and in some countries drastic measures are taken to enforce fertility control.

Both professionals and lay-people are becoming concerned about the unprecedented growth of populations, especially in the poorer continents of the world such as Africa and Asia.

The standard of living can be viewed as a scale. The balance between good and poor living standards is directly related to the various resources and means of life in a country on the one hand, and the population growth on the other hand. If the population growth is controlled and the resources found in a population are sufficient to provide for the needs of that population, there is a balance and optimal living conditions can be achieved within that population.

The resources of a population are its creative potential. However, not all people are in a position to contribute to the creative potential of the population. It is only a fraction of the population that is economically productive. The rest, for example those too old or too young to work and people with physical, mental or social disabilities who therefore cannot work and contribute economically to the population's creative potential, have to be supported by the country's resources, which are inversely related to the standard of living in that population.

In some developing countries the culture of a community may inhibit economic development as customs and values hinder the development of entrepreneurs or impede any decrease in fertility rates.

The consequences of uncontrolled fertility may have an adverse influence on the total well-being of the population. This can be depicted by the following formula:

$$\text{Standard of living} = \frac{\text{resources of the earth}}{\text{number of people who use resources}}$$

This formula suggests that the greater a country's resources, the higher its potential standard of living, but it also suggests that uncontrolled fertility adversely influences the economic, physical and psychological health of populations and family units, especially those existing at marginal and poverty levels.

FIGURE 4.2: A balanced optimal standard of living

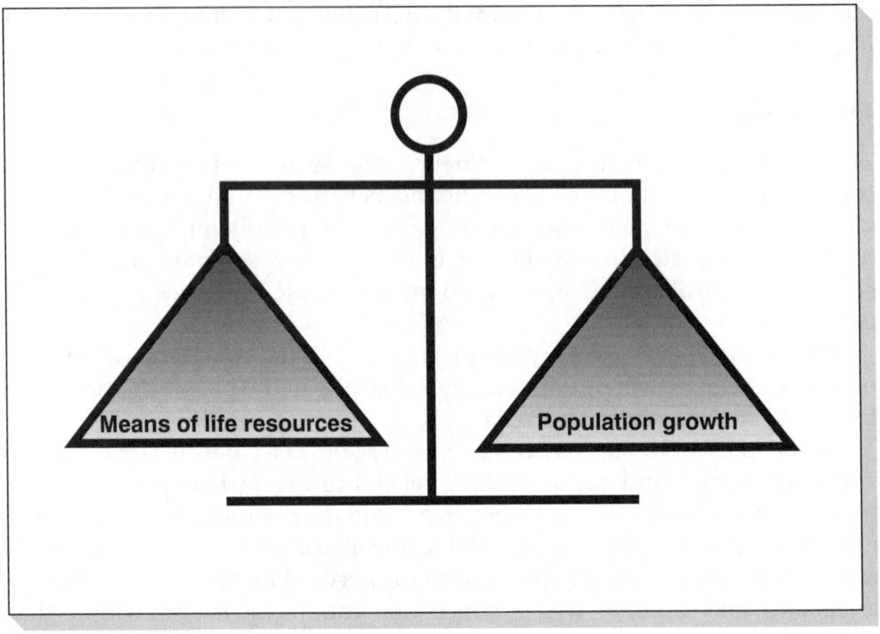

It can therefore be seen that the measurement of a country's fertility is extremely important in determining the optimal standard of living of its population, or in detecting the factors that may lead to a negative standard of living.

The measurement of fertility (or crude rate) has been described as a rough indicator of fertility. Everyone in the population, whether male, female, old or young, is taken into account when calculating the denominator. In terms of demography, however, more refined measures of fertility are needed, as not everyone in a population is regarded as fertile. Men, the aged and children cannot give birth and should therefore be excluded when determining the fertility rate in a population.

The denominator for the general fertility rate is restricted only to women of child-bearing age (15–49 years).

This general fertility rate is calculated as follows:

$$\text{General fertility rate} = \frac{\text{number of live births in an area in a specific year}}{\text{female population aged 15–49 years in same area in the same year}}$$

There are also other specific measures of fertility. These include the following:

- the age-specific fertility rate;
- the parity-specific fertility rate; and
- the age-parity-specific fertility rate.

FIGURE 4.3: Negative standard of living

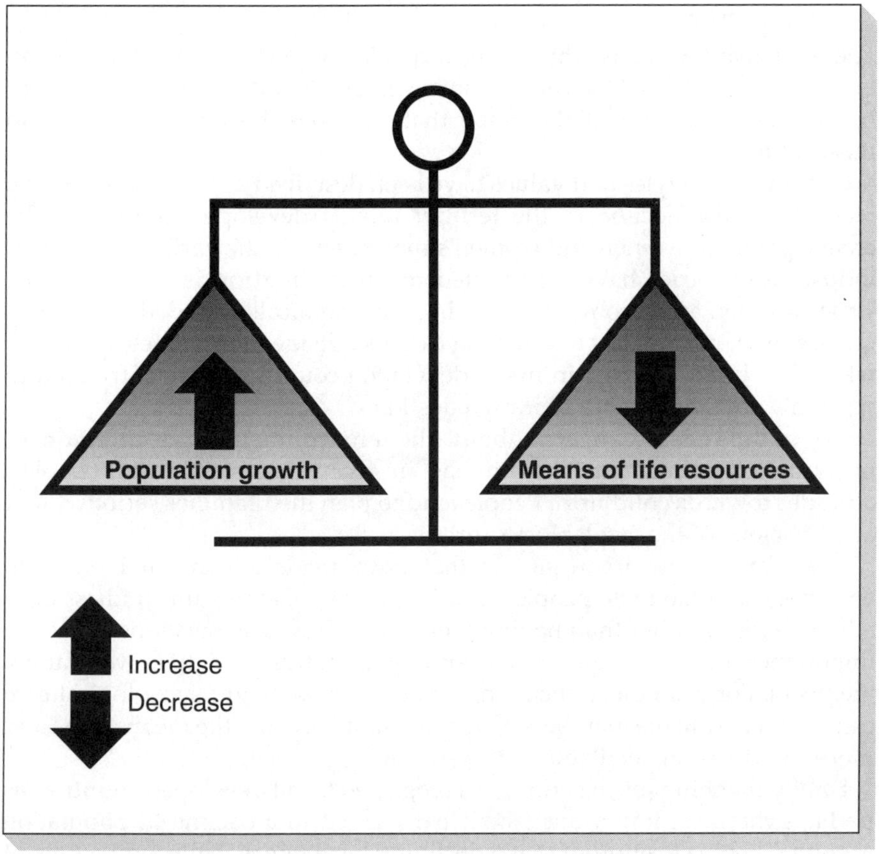

These calculations measure specific rates in a population. They are called period measures of fertility because they refer to births in a population over a specific period, usually a year, but other periods can also be used, such as a week, a month, ten years, etc. These rates are also calculated per 1 000, 10 000, 100 000, etc. of the population.

Another aspect of fertility is the cohort fertility rate. This is the fertility rate for women up to a certain age or during their "normal" productive years. A commonly used cohort measure of fertility is the completed birth rate – also called the final birth rate or completed fertility rate. This is defined as the number of children born per 1 000 women in a population by the end of their child-bearing period of 49 years (Mausner & Bahn 1974:214–215). For example, women might be delaying having their children during the expected child-bearing period of between 15 and 49 years of age because of a recession, war, violence or for other reasons.

4.8.1.1 *Possible reasons for the decline in fertility rates in developed countries*

There are many reasons why the fertility rate has declined over the years in developed countries. One cannot, however, single out only one reason, but has to take into account all the factors that could possibly have contributed to this decline.

Changing life-styles and values have been described as one of the possible reasons for the decline in the fertility rate in developed countries. The emancipation of women and women's movements in the various developed industrial countries have contributed much to the drop in the birth rate. Today women are becoming increasingly economically minded and active, qualifying in professions and having careers outside their homes. Abortion, which has been legalised in many developed countries, has contributed to women's decisions about their own destinies.

An enlightened concern about the environment and unplanned, uncontrolled population growth has in recent years changed people's attitudes towards childbirth. People tend to plan their families seriously and are conscious of the available resources.

There are many organisations that have made a concerted effort to encourage and motivate people to limit family size, to remain childless or to adopt children rather than having their own. These organisations stress the importance of giving qualitative and quantitative care to fewer family members. For example, education, health, nutrition and psychological care can be given to all the members of a small family because the means, time and money to do so are available.

Family planning (birth control) is recognised by all developed countries as perhaps the most important factor that has led to a decline in population growth. There is firm proof that a declining birth rate is really a direct result of safer and more readily available contraceptives.

Economic factors alone do not explain a decline in the birth rate in developed countries. We could rather focus on the changing attitudes of young people. They now seem to prefer to limit their family size to enjoy a higher standard of living and a fuller social life without the restrictions of having a large family.

4.8.1.2 *Fertility in developing countries*

In most developing countries there has been a sharp decline in the mortality rate and a sharp increase in the fertility rate. In Africa alone, the birth rate is estimated to be approaching 55 per 1 000 of the population and a decline in birth rates is not foreseen for the future.

The reasons for the difference between the fertility rates in developing and developed countries are as follows:

- The nations of the developing countries are not comparable to European or developed industrialised nations as they were several hundred years ago.

A decline in mortality in developed industrial countries occurred gradually over a period of several centuries. By contrast, the developing nations have shown a more rapid decline, primarily in the 20th century, because they applied westernised technology in, for example, the prevention, treatment and early detection of diseases.

- In developed countries this gradual decline in mortality was accompanied by considerable cultural and economic changes. In developing countries, however, the sudden decline in mortality has often been achieved without any major improvements in the living conditions, income, education, social change or economic development. Mortality decreases were actually the result of foreign influence and assistance.
- People in developing countries have limited ways of preventing either pregnancy or premature death - thus the aggregate population growth is rather low. However, as rudimentary medical care is introduced, the mortality rate often falls rapidly, while the higher fertility culture is maintained because children support parents in their old age and procreation is often a matter of tradition. This naturally leads to accelerated population growth and the population becomes increasingly younger.

Fertility decreases slowly as factors such as urbanisation, education, the need to provide adequately for children in terms of future education and even the increased availability of preventative health services and birth control make their presence felt. It is in this light that the South African population should be viewed, as each population group of this rainbow nation is in a different stage of demographic transition. This explains the differences in fertility, mortality, migration and therefore in morbidity.

4.8.1.3 Factors affecting the birth rate of a population

(a) Age at marriage

The average age at which women marry has an obvious effect on fertility. This age varies among different populations and is not a very objective measure in demography because there is a tendency among certain groups of people to bear children before they are married to show that they are fertile. Marriage is also a relative term, as certain traditional marriages are not regarded as legal forms of marriage in Western society.

(b) Biological factors

Biological factors may influence fertility, but this is not clearly understood. Some people live together, have normal sexual relations, but even without contraception seem to be infertile. It is also well known that certain nations are less and others more fertile.

(c) Birth control

Sterilisation in either males or females prevents conception without interfering with sexual activity, but is generally not accepted by large groups of people.

(d) Rural/urban differences

It is believed that people living in rural areas have higher fertility rates than those in urban areas. The larger the city, the lower the fertility. This is possibly because of the greater availability of work for women in larger cities. As they are probably more highly educated, they tend to have less time for large families and are more independent as professional people.

(e) Educational level and social status

Birth rates are higher among people who are poor and poorly educated than among those who are better educated and have a higher socio-economic status. It is also believed that the fertility is higher among blue-collar families than among white-collar families.

(f) Religion and culture

Catholics have a higher fertility than Protestants and the difference in Catholic-Protestant birth rates is growing. Black fertility is generally higher than white fertility, but in urban environments it follows white trends.

4.8.2 Mortality

The crude mortality rate is the number of deaths that have occurred in a specific year per 1 000 living persons in a specific population. It is determined partly by the health of the population and partly by its sex and age composition.

A population's death rate is affected by many factors, which may be cultural (e.g. sanitary practices), medical advancement and techniques, and the overall provision of health services in a country.

The infant mortality rate is the most significant component of the crude mortality rate, because the first year of life is the most vulnerable. In developing countries the number of infant deaths may exceed deaths in all other age groups.

It is through advanced technology and modernisation (factors that are often absent in developing countries) that mortality has been reduced. There are five interrelated factors that contribute to the reduction in mortality:

4.8.2.1 Improved medical technology

Improved medical technology in community health services and medical-care activities has led to an improvement in the disease rate and therefore in the death rate of a population. Immunisation and preventative measures have contributed to the eradication and prevention of various diseases such as smallpox. Infectious diseases such as tuberculosis, cholera and diphtheria are controlled by environmental measures and the elimination of rats, mosquitoes, lice and other factors has contributed to a healthier population.

The tracing and treatment of carriers of diseases such as syphilis has a great influence on the prevention and control of the spreading of disease.

The use of antibiotics, vaccines and antiseptics as well as the protection of food supplies from contamination leads to protection against diseases such as tuberculosis.

Advanced technology, applied in the timeous tracing of diseases such as cancer and in the long-term treatment of chronic diseases such as diabetes mellitus, heart conditions and surgical procedures, limits disabilities and ensures a longer, happier and healthier life.

4.8.2.2 *Improvement in living conditions*

There have been many changes in the living conditions in many countries of the world. This has contributed to a large reduction in the mortality rate of populations. People have become increasingly aware of the possibility of protection against the natural elements, for example by using air conditioning in warm areas and central heating in cold areas. With modern technology, water supplies, sanitation and hygiene are emphasised as some of the most important factors in the prevention of disease.

Improvements in the infrastructure of a population, for example transport facilities, education and communication, have made people aware of the necessity of exchanging knowledge on health matters and have led to a decline in the mortality rate.

4.8.2.3 *Improvement in the workplace*

Within the workplace many conditions previously led to exposure to harmful elements. Strict law enforcement to protect the workers from injuries and disease has ensured the safety and health of the work-force in the workplace. Workers have become more aware of the prevention of accidents, contamination from harmful substances and protective clothing. In general, better work conditions have led to the physical and mental well-being of workers.

Fatigue and over-exertion are prevented through better working hours, rest periods and vacations. There are restrictions on the age of the work-force and special care is taken of children, the aged and vulnerable workers. Women in the workplace are protected during pregnancy and special care is taken of the unborn baby.

4.8.2.4 *Improvement of maternity and child-care facilities*

Many improvements have been made to the childbearing and child-care conditions which, in turn, have considerably limited maternity and infant mortality. Free or cheap contraceptives are available for all who want them to reduce the number of pregnancies that are either unwanted or ill-timed for the family. Dangerous cultural practices have not been eliminated altogether, but have to a great extent been taken care of in traditional societies.

4.8.2.5 *Improved nutrition*

The improvement of nutrition is an important factor in the decline of mortality, especially in the developing countries. Nutritional supplements such as high-protein supplements, powdered baby foods and vitamin tablets have contributed to better standards of nutrition in many countries.

There are, however, still countries (e.g. Ethiopia) where famine and malnutrition are rife. These conditions can be due to political disputes, acts of terrorism, unrest, natural disasters (such as droughts) or to an exceedingly high population growth where sufficient food can no longer be produced to sustain the population.

4.8.3 Migration

Migration is a change of residence in which a recognised boundary of some type is crossed, for example if a person decides to move to a different country, a different province, or from an urban to a rural area. It is regarded as the rate at which people in a community or country move into (immigrate to) or out of (emigrate from) a society. The difference between immigration and emigration during a given period, for example one year, is termed a population's "net migration".

International migration accounts for only a small fraction of the world population figures. Migrants are unevenly distributed among countries. For some countries, demographic change is an important economic factor. The 1980s witnessed the resurgence of international migration as a worldwide phenomenon, with widening gaps between countries in terms of demographic growth and economic progress.

This phenomenon can occur because of certain "push factors" such as unemployment, food shortages and racial or religious discrimination, or because of certain "pull factors" such as cheap land, availability of jobs, better living conditions or the prospect of making money.

International migration takes place across international borders and can be an important factor which may bring about drastic changes within a particular area.

Migration may have far-reaching consequences for a community or a country as a whole, which may be positive as well as negative:

- it may provide a cheap source of labour;
- it may contribute to the increased population size of a country or community;
- the concept of the "melting pot" is implied – it is an important way of enriching and diversifying the cultural heritage of a community;

- technology can be enriched;
- greater opportunities for employment are created;
- refugees send home much-needed money and goods to care for their families who have been left behind; and
- it provides labour and expands markets.

It may, however, have negative consequences for the community because it may put greater pressure on resources such as housing, water, food supply and medical care. There is also greater job competition and migrants put a strain on the economy as more houses, schools, educational facilities and infrastructures must be provided. Refugees or immigrants may also bring with them foreign diseases which had been hitherto unknown in a population. The local population may not have developed any resistance to the disease and could be seriously affected.

Returning refugees may bring back a new life-style, which may affect the lives of those who were left behind. This new life-style could have either positive or negative consequences, or it may increase their hopes for the future for their children.

Whether migrants remain in the foreign country, return to their native land for visits, or return as permanent residents, they are powerful agents of change in a population.

The current trends in internal migration are the shifts from rural to urban areas, from central cities to suburbs and from inland to coastal areas. South Africa also has refugees from other African countries who, for political or economic reasons, migrate to this country. This tendency may have a massive impact on the total structure of a community and a country as a whole. It puts a strain on the provision of all facilities, health services and the personnel who are required to meet health needs.

In South Africa, migrant workers contribute to the change in the demography of the country. Migrant workers are people without a fixed residence who are mainly, but not necessarily, engaged in agriculture, mining and seasonal industries. One can also include military troops and college or university students who have two residences and who only migrate for a particular purpose to a certain area for a specific period of time. Among vagrants there is a shift from one area to another as the seasons change. It is impossible for a country to get definite numbers in respect of these migratory groups. This can be a serious handicap to health planners and other public officials in the planning of services, such as the provision of housing, water and recreation facilities.

4.8.4 The composition of the South African population

South Africa is a distinctly diverse, plural and dynamic nation. Its composition shows this distinctive character.

4.8.4.1 The total composition

Statistical data can never be completed or updated to the last moment of the last birth or death. Even as you read this chapter, the composition of the population is changing. Estimates are given, as they are at least data we can to use to get a picture of the composition and characteristics of the population of a country.

The various races are given separately, as different races may be seen to have different needs. Cultures and epidemiological patterns differ among the different races. It is a natural population characteristic that is typical of humans and therefore an essential aspect of differentiation in demographic terms. Affiliation to a specific population sector involves typical living situations but also stress situations that expose members of that group to certain risk factors to a greater or lesser degree.

It is estimated that in 1994, the South African population numbered some 40,4 million people. Of these 76 per cent were black, 8,5 per cent coloured, 2,6 per cent Indian and 12,8 per cent white.

Table 4.1 shows the total composition of the South African population in 1994, by province. The exclusion of the former homelands renders the reliability of the data questionable. It is, however, an important indicator for nurses about the total fertility rate, which assists them in planning and predicting future needs for services.

TABLE 4.1 The racial composition and growth rate of the South African population in 1994

Racial group	Number	% of population	Crude birth rate	Crude death rate	Average annual growth rate %
Black	30 767 300	76,1	25,3	10,2	2,5
Coloured	3 449 000	8,5	21,7	7,2	1,5
Indian	1 035 000	2,6	18,1	7,3	1,5
White	5 184 000	12,8	13,7	6,7	0,7
Total South Africa	**40 435 300**	**100**	**23,4**	**9,4**	**2,1**

Source: Central Statistical Services (1994)

Table 4.3 depicts the age and sex distribution of the South African population in 1991. It shows that:

- there are slightly more females than males;
- the black population is quite young, with over 25% of the population being below 15 years of age;
- the median for blacks is 22,4 years in contrast with that of the white population, which is much older;
- the white population is ageing, with 9,4% of the population in the age group 65 years and older; and

TABLE 4.2: The basic structure of the South African population by race in 1991				
	Racial group			
Characteristic	**Black**	**Coloured**	**Indian**	**White**
% Female	5,2	51,6	50,7	50,9
% Male	48,8	48,4	49,3	49,1
% aged 0–4	11,1	10,5	8,7	7,2
% aged 5–14	23,2	22,3	20,9	16,3
% aged 15–64	61,8	63,7	67,2	67,2
% aged 65+	3,8	3,6	3,1	9,4
Sex ratio (M/F)	95,3	93,7	97,1	96,0
Median aged	22,4	23,0	24,8	30,9

Source: Central Statistical Services (1994)

- the percentage of the population in the economically active ages is smaller for blacks and coloureds than for whites and Indians.

Age and sex distribution are important for the nurse with regard to the planning of services and the prediction of disease patterns. The various age and sex groups have different needs and in the South African health care system much is done for the mothers and children of the country.

TABLE 4.3: Age and sex distribution of the South African population by racial group in 1991								
	Racial group							
Age group	**Black**		**Coloured**		**Indian**		**White**	
	M	**F**	**M**	**F**	**M**	**F**	**M**	**F**
0–4	11,3	10,9	10,8	10,2	9,0	8,4	7,4	6,9
5–9	12,1	11,5	12,0	11,2	10,8	10,1	8,5	8,9
10–14	11,5	11,3	11,2	10,3	10,8	10,2	8,5	7,7
15–19	10,5	10,9	11,3	10,5	11,3	10,8	9,3	8,7
20–24	9,8	10,4	10,5	10,4	9,7	9,5	8,5	8,3
25–29	9,4	9,4	9,2	9,5	8,5	8,9	7,9	7,8
30–34	8,9	8,2	8,1	8,4	8,0	8,3	8,1	7,9
35–39	6,6	6,1	6,5	6,8	7,3	7,3	7,5	7,3
40–44	5,5	5,1	5,3	5,6	6,8	7,0	7,2	7,0
45–49	3,9	3,6	4,0	4,2	5,5	5,5	6,2	6,0
50–54	3,2	3,2	3,5	3,6	4,2	4,4	5,3	5,2
55–59	2,1	2,3	2,6	2,8	2,9	3,1	4,2	4,3
60–64	1,8	2,6	1,9	2,3	2,2	2,6	3,7	4,1
65–69	1,2	1,6	1,3	1,6	1,4	1,6	2,9	3,5
70–74	1,1	1,4	0,8	0,9	0,8	0,9	2,2	2,9
75–79	0,4	0,6	0,4	0,5	0,4	0,5	1,4	2,2
80+	0,5	0,7	0,3	0,4	0,3	0,4	1,1	2,4

Source: Development Bank (1995:22–3)

TABLE 4.4: The racial distribution of the provincial population in 1994				
	Racial group (%)			
Province	**Black**	**Coloured**	**Indian**	**White**
Western Cape	17,4	57,8	0,8	24,0
Eastern Cape	87,3	6,9	0,0	5,8
Northern Cape	31,7	51,9	0,0	16,2
Free State	84,0	2,7	0,0	13,3
KwaZulu-Natal	82,1	1,2	9,5	7,2
North-West	90,7	1,4	0,0	7,9
Gauteng	62,7	4,1	2,2	31,1
Mpumalanga	88,9	0,5	0,4	10,2
Northern Province	97,0	0,1	0,1	2,8

Source: Development Bank (1995:22–3)

Table 4.4 shows the racial distribution of the South African population per province in 1994. The distribution of the population among the nine provinces clearly indicates the former labour, employment and demographic policies, which were racially determined.

TABLE 4.5: The percentage of the South African population in each province, provincial population density and urbanisation status in 1994			
Province	**% of total population**	**Population density (per/km^2)**	**% urban**
Western Cape	9,0	28,1	86,4
Eastern Cape	16,1	38,0	32,8
Northern Cape	1,9	2,0	73,1
Free State	6,9	21,1	54,1
KwaZulu-Natal	21,2	92,3	38,2
North-West	8,3	28,0	32,2
Gauteng	17,0	365,2	96,0
Mpumalanga	7,2	37,3	31,6
Northern Province	12,4	42,2	9,2
South Africa	100	33,0	48,8

Source: Development Bank (1995:121–53)

4.8.4.2 The fertility rate of the South African population

The fertility rate of the South African population in 1990 is depicted in Table 4.7. Blacks have the largest families and whites the smallest. A rough fertility measure is the average number of children per woman past childbearing age (over the age of 49). Orieji Chimere-Dan (1995:10) concludes that, although it gives an indication of the fertility level, this measure should be carefully interpreted. It is a cohort measure that does not

TABLE 4.6: Average household size by province and racial group in 1990					
	Racial group				
Province	**Black**	**Coloured**	**Indian**	**White**	**All**
Western Cape	3,9	4,8	—	3,0	3,9
Eastern Cape	5,3	5,5	—	3,7	5,2
Northern Cape	3,5	4,5	—	—	4,3
Free State	4,0	3,5	—	3,1	3,9
KwaZulu-Natal	6,2	4,4	4,5	2,6	5,7
North-West	3,9	—	—	3,1	3,8
Gauteng	3,8	4,4	4,4	3,0	3,5
Mpumalanga	4,7	—	—	3,5	4,6
Northern Province	5,4	—	—	2,5	5,2
Rural	5,1	4,8	—	3,2	5,1
Urban	4,3	4,7	4,4	3,0	4,0
South Africa	4,8	4,7	4,4	3,0	4,5

Source: University of Cape Town (1994)

capture the experiences of all woman of reproductive age. Quite often it is affected by the small number of woman used in the calculation of the statistics. It is best used together with fertility rate to assess trends in fertility.

In South Africa, as in all the other developing countries, the fertility of the country is the most widely studied component of population dynamics, as it influences the total structure of the economy and all other development aspects in a country.

TABLE 4.7: The total fertility rate of the South African population in 1990					
	Racial group				
Province	**Black**	**Coloured**	**Indian**	**White**	**Total**
Western Cape	4,4	2,9	2,7	1,5	2,8
Eastern Cape	4,4	3,1	2,4	1,6	4,1
Northern Cape	4,1	3,1	2,8	2,0	3,6
Free State	2,8	2,2	2,1	1,8	2,7
KwaZulu-Natal	2,2	2,8	2,3	1,5	2,2
North-West	3,5	2,0	1,8	1,9	3,3
Gauteng	2,6	2,8	2,6	1,8	2,4
Mpumalanga	3,7	2,4	2,1	2,1	3,5
Northern Province	5,7	2,6	2,2	2,4	5,6
South Africa (1990)	3,7	2,7	2,3	1,8	3,3

Source: Department of National Health and Population Development (1993)

The values given in the last row of Table 4.8 show completed family sizes for women aged 45 to 49 by race. The average growth rate for whites fluctuated and declined sharply to the lowest of all four population groups. The annual growth rate of the black population shows a marked higher growth rate than

TABLE 4.8: The average number of children per woman of reproductive age in South Africa, by age and racial group in 1993

Age group	Racial group				
	Black	Coloured	Indian	White	South Africa
15–19	0,2	0,1	0,0	0,0	0,1
20–24	0,9	0,5	0,4	0,3	0,8
25–29	1,8	1,5	1,2	1,0	1,7
30–34	2,8	2,6	2,3	1,7	2,6
35–39	3,7	3,1	2,5	2,4	3,4
40–44	4,4	3,8	2,8	2,3	3,9
45–49	5,0	4,2	3,0	2,5	4,3

Source: University of Cape Town (1994)

TABLE 4.9: Estimates of life expectation at birth for provinces by race and sex in 1990

Province	Racial group									
	Black		Coloured		Indian		White		All	
	M	F	M	F	M	F	M	F	M	F
Western Cape	60	65	59	66	62	64	70	78	63	68
Eastern Cape	59	64	55	62	61	74	68	76	61	68
Northern Cape	60	65	57	61	56	59	69	76	60	65
Free State	60	65	69	61	—		69	75	61	66
KwaZulu-Natal	61	66	62	70	63	69	70	76	62	69
North-West	63	68	65	65	65	70	68	76	64	70
Gauteng	64	69	59	66	67	72	69	75	63	69
Mpumalanga	61	66	61	70	63	69	68	77	63	69
Northern Province	59	64	62	70	62	69	70	77	62	68
South Africa	60	67	50	65	64	70	69	76	62	68

Source: University of Cape Town (1993)

that of the other three race groups. The annual growth rate for coloureds declined, as did that of the Asian population.

Table 4.9 shows the estimates of expected live births by race and sex in the different provinces of South Africa. The data should however be viewed with extreme caution and it should be remembered that only estimates are given. These data exclude the former TBVC states.

The following aspects can be highlighted:

- infant mortality rates for blacks are higher in the Northern Province, Mpumalanga and the Free State;
- the highest level of infant mortality rates for coloureds and whites are in the Free State; and
- Indians have their highest mortality rate in KwaZulu-Natal.

The implications of sexually transmitted diseases and HIV/AIDS for the infant mortality rate has caused considerable concern, but thus far there are no reliable statistics to substantiate the influence of these factors on the infant mortality rate.

Ideally, a comprehensive and reliable national census with extended health and mortality questions will provide good basic demographic data for contextualised modelling and discussion of the demographic impact of HIV/AIDS on the South African population.

TABLE 4.10: Projected growth of the South African population (millions)

Year	Total population	Asians	Blacks	Coloureds	Whites
Low fertility assumptions					
1990	39,506	0,959	30,289	3,237	5,021
2000	51,173	1,096	40,966	3,805	5,307
2010	64,381	1,203	53,375	4,273	5,529
2020	76,996	1,309	65,308	4,681	5,697
2030	89,083	1,385	76,833	5,110	5,755
2035	94,380	1,410	81,943	5,273	5,754
High fertility assumptions					
1990	39,527	0,961	30,289	3,245	5,031
2000	51,420	1,108	41,044	3,856	5,413
2010	66,542	1,235	55,155	4,417	5,736
2020	85,219	1,355	72,943	4,947	5,975
2030	107,076	1,445	94,051	5,454	6,126
2035	118,881	1,479	105,566	5,665	6,171

Source: Marais (1988:80)

TABLE 4.11: Immigration and emigration in South Africa in 1992–1994

	1994	1993	1992
Immigrants	6 398	9 824	8 686
Emigrants	10 235	8 078	4 289
Net	−3 837	+746	+4 397

Source: Central Statistical Services (1994)

The immigration and emigration figures for South Africa are shown in Table 4.11. The data do not include undocumented or illegal immigrants, refugees and asylum seekers, whose numbers in South Africa appear to be increasing rapidly following the full integration of the country into the international community. In most cases, their numbers can only be guessed at.

4.9 THE CONSEQUENCES OF RAPID POPULATION GROWTH

4.9.1 Age structure and economic development

The combination of low mortality and high fertility is a typical phenomenon of developing countries that tend to have a very young age structure. In developing countries it is also recognised that the highest rate of mortality occurs among infants and children. It is also noted by many authors that in all the developing countries 40 to 50 per cent of the population is younger than 15 years of age. This puts the economy and the health services of a country under strain, as the young people in the population consume more than they produce. In societies where there is a young age structure, few resources are available for investment in economic development. Most resources are simply used for day-to-day living for those who cannot provide for themselves.

There are many problems associated with this very young age structure, for example:

- Educational and training facilities, skilled personnel and the infrastructure for education and training must be provided to accommodate this specific age structure.
- Jobs and opportunities have to be provided – young people want to achieve something in life, they have high hopes and are motivated. In a developing country with a declining economy, the provision of jobs is not always possible. As a result, there are many retrenchments of older people to make place for the younger generation and there is strong competition for jobs and opportunities.
- An economic burden is placed on the governing body of a country as well as on the taxpayer to provide facilities and services for this generation of young people that does not provide for itself.
- Health services are especially influenced by the growth of the younger generation and services have to be supplied, skilled personnel trained and large sums of money spent on needs specifically associated with a young age group.

One of the major consequences of the decline in fertility is the number of older people in the population. This is a typical tendency in developed countries. The age structure affects both its potential productivity and the health needs in a community. A society with a large number of old people may have many problems, such as:

- increased medical costs;
- an increased demand for trained medical, nursing and social services personnel;
- unproductive sectors of the population because of the age and declining physical health of groups of individuals; a responsibility is placed on the

state and therefore on the taxpayer to provide for those who are unproductive; and

- residential and other services have to be supplied.

It was disclosed by Mostert *et al.* in Marais (1988:84) that a sharp increase in the elderly is expected among all the population groups of South Africa but more so amongst the Asian, white and coloured population groups.

It is estimated that there are globally more than 1 billion people who are living in absolute poverty. The total international debt of developing countries is currently $1 200 billion and that figure is still growing.

The social sector, including health, family planning, housing and education, continue to be emphasised in national and international development programmes. At national level, developing countries such as South Africa are struggling to keep pace with the needs of the population, which have often doubled in the last 30 years. The demands for health care, housing, jobs, education, food and security are increasing and will continue to increase throughout the next decade and beyond.

4.9.2 Urbanisation and urban growth

Urbanisation and urban growth is a problem connected with rapid population growth in developing countries. Urbanisation tends to take place without corresponding social change. Services and facilities cannot keep up with this phenomenon and therefore social problems occur.

It can be said that the developing world (including South Africa) is in the middle of an urban revolution, fuelled in part by massive population shifts from rural to urban areas. It is said that by the year 2000, over half of humanity will live in urban areas. Certain cities will reach gigantic proportions in the near future. Balancing rural and urban development strategies is likely to prove to be a tough and delicate process in national and provincial policies in the near future.

Given the rapid and largely unplanned urbanisation, there is concern that in the developing world the abilities of municipalities are not keeping up with demand for infrastructure and services. In many cities of developing countries, the demand for housing, roads, health care, educational facilities and the provision of commodities such as safe drinking water, electricity and sanitation have outpaced the supply and drastic measures will have to be taken to upgrade these facilities to keep up with the rising tide of urban inhabitants.

There is a large pool of unemployed, underemployed, unskilled and semi-skilled labour that is the consequence of the rising urban population. These people often land up in slums and squatter settlements and a vicious circle of unemployment, lack of education, undernourishment and chronic illnesses continues to grow. Thousands of people end their days in the streets where they are found in shelters of makeshift shacks, fashioned from discarded wood, canvas and cardboard. These people become permanently marginalised and caught up in a vicious circle of poverty.

Surveys of squatter camps have found that many of the residents have lived in them for more than a decade. There is neither upward nor downward mobility. They begin their lives poor and end them poor, passing it on to the next generation who, in turn, continue to live their lives on the margins of survival. It should be recognised that the same situation often prevails in rural areas where most of the poor throughout the world are concentrated.

One of the biggest concerns of the alarming rapid rate of urbanisation is the loss of prime arable agricultural land. Many hectares of crop and grazing land are being taken up to build houses, industrial areas, refuse dumps, graveyards and buildings for offices, flats etc.

4.9.3 Demand for resources

Population growth poses a threat to the survival of the nations in the developing countries. It puts an increasing strain on the available resources. Population growth is one of the most significant factors to undermine the environmental resources. In many countries (including Southern African countries) there is a pronounced imbalance between the growth of the population on the one hand and the natural resources that must support it.

There are some prominent population factors that are regarded by many of the foremost authors as serious concerns for their significant impact on resource depletion and their influence on environmental quality. They include:

4.9.3.1 Loss of agricultural land

This issue has already been dealt with in terms of rapid urbanisation, but it should be noted that if land gets more worn out by continuous crop production and erosion, it gets degraded to such an extent that crop production is no longer possible and that it no longer can be used for grazing. It is estimated that 70 000 square kilometres of farm land in the world are abandoned because the soil gets degraded to such an extent that no crops can be ever produced on these lands. Another 200 000 square kilometres suffer from reduced productivity and there is little hope for their recovery.

The most gloomy pictures painted are those of the extent of land degradation in soil erosion. This claims 24 billion tons of topsoil in the world every year.

4.9.3.2 The concentration of population in critical ecological zones

The concentration of large groups of people in the sensitive ecological zones of the world, including South Africa, is cause for concern. Climate, the sea, the availability of food and other attractions for humans contribute to migration to ecologically sensitive areas, where within a short time they deplete the natural resources, pollute and mostly change the ecological balance that has existed for millions of years.

4.9.3.3 *The destruction of tropical forests*

The World Bank has recently estimated that 17–20 million hectares of tropical forests are destroyed annually. This deforestation is taking place in developing countries. The reasons are:

- encroachment by landless slash-and-burn cultivators;
- large-scale logging operations; and
- conversion of grazing land to large plantations.

The major underlying driving forces of the destruction of tropical forests are rural poverty and population growth. Migrant populations in forested areas in Southern Africa have increased rapidly over the last decade and with this comes the destruction of sensitive forests.

The accessibility of remote wilderness and coastal areas, for example the breeding places of many rare and sensitive species, have caused an increase in the population density there and with the pressure to intensify cultivation, increase harvests and to gather forest products such as rare plants (e.g. the precious and rare cycads found in KwaZulu-Natal and the Cape), settlements have expanded to remote and steeper locations.

Forest resources are depleted more rapidly than they can be replaced, for example through the harvesting of tree bark and scarce indigenous plants for traditional use. The collection of dry wood for fires depletes the soil of essential nutrients that can never be replaced. Furthermore, the fuel to cook meals comes from trees. There are many rural areas where trees are being cut off or branches are being removed one by one, leaving the soil barren.

Where forests are converted to farms, the serious consequences may be seen in the severity of flooding often experienced. Top soil is washed away and soil erosion occurs where there is no grass cover or natural protection. The stones, rocks and gravel that protect the ground and prevent erosion are often removed to build roads and houses, or used as filling for other eroded areas, leaving the soil vulnerable to erosion.

4.9.3.4 *Freshwater resources*

Excessive population growth is occurring in many countries that may be regarded as poor as far as their water resources are concerned. An even more alarming factors is that the limited water resources in these countries are also polluted. Water pollution, however, is not only a problem in developing countries, but also in developed countries. Degraded water quality directly affects human health and welfare, while it indirectly contributes to slower rates of development.

Water-related land degradation threatens the sustainable use of resources. This is a particular problem in areas dependent on irrigated agriculture, where salination, water-logging and alkalisation are turning once productive cropland into wasteland. Furthermore, salts released from irrigated soils are polluting surface waters.

There are four basic types of water scarcity:

- Inter-annual fluctuations in some areas, which result in recurrent droughts with large areas of unproductive soil. South Africa has just been through a time of severe drought and is known for fluctuations in the rain pattern, therefore predictions of good rainfall are never reliable. In rainy seasons, severe floods wash away precious soil and ground cover to rivers and dams, causing obstruction and flooding and the breaking of walls and dams. Water scarcity then still remains a problem as the resources to store water have been washed away.
- Desiccation of the landscape, such as large-scale deforestation, the destruction of watersheds and overgrazing of grasslands are evident throughout Southern Africa. Such activities strip away the natural vegetation that not only protects soil against torrential rains, but that is necessary for human existence. Massive soil erosion causes fertile lands to become unproductive and water to run off before it can recharge rivers and aquifers or even be captured for other uses.
- Water evaporation is so rapid that aquifers and rivers cannot be recharged. This is typical of deserts and arids, which are a growing problem in some areas in Southern Africa.
- Perhaps the greatest concern, i.e. water scarcity, is due to an increasing demand by the ever-growing population and its grossly inefficient use of water resources. This is one of the biggest threats to human existence.

In essence, the combination of land degradation and intermittent droughts, as found in almost all the areas of Southern Africa, increases the risk of crop failures, which in turn lead to famine. Population growth aggravates this problem because there is less water *per capita* to support human life, to improve health and food security and to increase market-orientated activities such as cash crops and industrial production.

Water scarcity already affects 88 developing countries and 40 per cent of the world population. Without a worldwide water policy, many severe crises will arise that may threaten further industrial development and the expansion of agriculture. This poses a serious threat to human existence.

4.9.3.5 Loss of biological diversity

Tropical forests continue to disappear as a result of rapid population growth and industrialisation. A wealth of flora and fauna with genetic resources of inestimable value to human welfare have already been lost and are disappearing every day.

It is estimated by the foundations that protect and monitor wildlife and plants that 10 to 30 million plant and animal species exist. Clearing forests and natural lands may eliminate thousands of species, which are lost forever. As the human species increases, other species decrease.

4.9.3.6 *Climatic change*

There is concern about climatic changes caused by emissions of the so-called "green-house gases". Recent research confirms the build-up of green-house gases in the atmosphere. It is estimated that carbon dioxide levels have risen from 2,4 billion tons in 1950 to 6,8 billion tons in 1985. They are increasing at a minimum rate of 3,1 per cent per annum. During the same period an average population growth of 1,9 per cent was reported. Population growth is responsible for almost two thirds of the increase in carbon dioxide emissions.

The link between population growth and climate changes is basically twofold:

- Through population growth a higher *per capita* energy consumption level is demanded. This demand for energy, power, industry and transport leads to wastes in the atmosphere in which carbon is deposited.
- Population growth causes deforestation, which is associated with emissions of carbon dioxide. Cutting down trees, and burning grass and plants reduces the mayor land-based sink for carbon dioxide.

4.9.3.7 *Pollution*

Pollution of the land, soil, water and air is evidence of man's existence on earth. Drastic measures will have to be taken by all countries and greater efforts should by made by South Africa's population and authorities to ensure the continued survival of mankind. Pollution takes many forms and has a devastating influence on every form of life on earth.

4.10 LIFESPAN AND LIFE EXPECTANCY

Modernisation has brought about a higher life expectancy for the world population and early mortality is prevented - people tend to die of old age or age-related diseases. Life expectancy is a demographic factor that is closely linked to a population's mortality and morbidity. It is observed that most developing societies have relatively high birth rates, high death rates and as a result of these also a reasonable young population. In addition, these societies also have a low life expectancy. The typical disease pattern is that of acute infections as a result of infectious diseases. It is thus not typical for these people to develop chronic diseases - because too few people live long enough to develop them. As the life expectancy rises, the disease pattern changes and more chronic diseases are found.

The lifespan of an individual is regarded as the maximum age that a person can reach in his life under favourable conditions until he ultimately dies of old age, while life expectancy is an estimate of the average length of life.

The available data indicate that a high life expectancy is characterised by populations in developed societies and communities. It can therefore be concluded that as a society's level of development increases, the life expectancy of the population will show a corresponding upward trend.

4.11 DEMOGRAPHIC TRENDS AND THEIR INFLUENCE ON HEALTH AND NURSING

An increased population places a great demand on the health-care services, with a concomitant shortage of qualified personnel to care for the needs of the population.

Population increases mean an increasing demand for food and sources of energy, and this leads to the soaring costs of these means of life. Many low-income families have to endure hunger, extremes of temperature, poor living conditions and facilities that are detrimental to their physical and mental well-being.

Higher life expectancy places demands on care, facilities and trained personnel. With an increasingly ageing population, great emphasis is placed on the prevention, diagnosis and treatment of chronic diseases, which have great economic consequences for the state as well as for the individual. Large numbers of adolescents in a community, on the other hand, place an increasing emphasis on the control of sexually transmitted diseases such as AIDS, teenage pregnancy, educational programmes, abortion and contraceptives.

Social problems that must be dealt with in a growing society include drug abuse, child neglect and abuse, alcoholism, suicide and family disintegration.

Health-care services have to provide for both the young and the old, requiring nurses to be able to meet the needs of people in various age groups and to assist them in achieving their optimal developmental potential and health.

Urbanisation and its associated problems influence the health of individuals and families, not only on a physical level, but also mentally with the increase of stress-related diseases, neuroses, etc. Urbanisation has resulted in social problems such as vagrants and street children, and in political instability in high-density residential areas.

With urbanisation comes a decrease in the availability of support systems and this places a great responsibility on the nurse to assist the client to develop alternative support systems and coping mechanisms to face rapid social change.

In South Africa there is no official policy on population. The previous government emphasised the reduction of fertility and in 1984 a Population

Development Programme was established to provide contraceptive services and to create public awareness of the importance of fertility reduction.

Since 1993 there have been important developments and changes in population polices and activities in South Africa. The authorities have defined new directions for population programmes with the full involvement of interested institutions.

The population policy and programmes are sensitive issues that cannot be changed overnight by politicians and policymakers. To substantiate concrete arguments, reliable demographic data are needed. Nurses can make a contribution in this regard.

South Africa has been admitted into the World Health arena after centuries of isolation.

In 1994 the United Nations Population Fund, the main UN body responsible for population activities, resumed operations in South Africa. It remains to be seen whether the return of the international community in general and the United Nations Fund for Population Activities (UNFPA) in particular will facilitate communication among policymakers who presently hold diverging views on population policy and programmes in the country.

4.12 A POPULATION EXPLOSION

The causes of population growth are extremely complex and one cannot predict the future population growth with any certainty. A high population rate conjures up spectres of large-scale poverty, unemployment and general overburdening of the existing infrastructure. Population growth and economic performance can be regarded as two sides of the same coin, both having negative and positive effects on one another.

On the one hand a large, well-educated population can provide the production factor labour in the production process. On the other hand it can consume the efforts of production, causing devastation.

An adequate supply of young, educated and productive workers may generate sufficient income, taxes and trade to pay the pensions of the previous generation, those that cannot care for themselves and to secure the future for the next generation.

With a growing economy that stimulates adequate health care, education and financial security, the need for larger families may decrease which, in return, results in lower population growth.

The capacity of the earth to support this increasingly growing population is seriously in question and the present growth cannot be indefinitely maintained.

Cultural and psychological factors are associated with high fertility and, although family planning measures have been introduced in nearly all the countries of the world and abortion is legally available in many countries, there is still an increasing rate of fertility.

The principal reasons for the failure of birth control seem to be the following:

- the ignorance and isolation of young women;
- a lack of communication between husbands and their wives on sexual matters;
- attitudes of certain cultures and religious groups towards family planning and contraception;
- the fear of the atmosphere and practices at family-planning clinics;
- the dependency and timidity of women in relation to their husbands;
- the high value that men place on large families, particularly male (or, in certain cultures, female) children as symbols of their virility;
- the misconception that children will provide for the parents in their old age; and
- the view that many children mean prosperity.

Past population studies concentrated the attention too narrowly on fertility and how it can be reduced. The consistent downward trend in the total fertility rate for all racial groups discourages the adoption of a policy that places exclusive and heavy emphasis on fertility reduction. The existing evidence on demographic development points to wider dimensions of the population issue that were ignored in the past. These include infant mortality, migration, rural and urban development, inequality in the access to national resources, the social and legal position of women and aspects of reproductive health that have strong links to demographic processes. A national population policy should therefore be more broadly conceived and rooted in the historical experiences and contemporary basic needs of the South African population.

4.13 TOWARDS ZERO POPULATION GROWTH

Zero population growth is a state of equilibrium that is seen by many as the essential goal if the human race is to avoid over-abusing the capacity of the environment to feed and to support the nations of the world.

It means that parents should strive to have children only to replace themselves – thus two children per family. In the United States and in many countries in Europe, this goal has already been achieved.

Replacement levels should ideally be maintained for a period of at least 25 years before zero population growth is actually attained.

4.14 RECOMMENDATIONS FOR SOLVING DEMOGRAPHIC PROBLEMS

Demographic changes such as the patterns of development, environmental degradation and population growth and distribution are reaching critical proportions in most of the developing world. There is therefore an urgent need to address the problem, as human existence depends on prompt action. The following recommendations are made:

- Population growth must be minimised. The avoidable part of population growth should be mitigated by child spacing. Emphasis must be placed on the promotion of a small, healthy family. To achieve this, great emphasis should be placed on popular education and participation, especially on the part of women. Nurses are in the unique position that they can educate, motivate and encourage people in their communities to ensure that a better quality of life can be attained by child spacing and population management.
- Governments are urged to establish or strengthen mechanisms to coordinate policies and programmes and to give unified direction for integrating environmental and population concerns into development policy making and planning. Nurses have the benefit that they act as leaders in their communities. They must use their skills, knowledge and influence to make leaders aware of problems and to establish programmes for the benefit of the communities.
- The government is urged fully to take into account the implications of the projected demographic trends and patterns of production and consumption. Policy, facts and/or figures often exist on paper alone, while nothing is seriously being done. The seriousness of the problems should be taken into account by top government officials and policy makers.
- The conservation of natural resources should be of the utmost importance and national conservation strategies must be formulated.
- The balance between population growth and resources must be maintained. It is the responsibility of the government to support and develop technology to achieve sustained economic growth and development.
- Developed countries should make technology available to developing countries at a reasonable cost. International assistance and collaboration is of the utmost importance.
- Environmental conditions should be improved and further environmental degradation should at all costs be avoided. Governments should identify sensitive areas such as coastal regions, which are subject to acute population pressures, and develop policies that will alleviate the pressure on the environment.
- Governments and the private sector should work hand in hand to implement ecologically beneficial, labour-intensive projects such as reforestation, contour-levelling, terracing, irrigation and proper and efficient drainage for environmental benefits, as well as assisting in job creation to prevent exploitation of the environment.
- Women are the backbone of every community. It is essential that they should participate in community-based population and environmental

programmes. Women can contribute to conservation programmes, as well as the reforestation, conservation and development of parks and protected areas. It is therefore essential that women's educational level, health status, employment opportunities, environmental sensitivity and participation in all decision-making bodies must be encouraged.

- It is a fact that some areas in the Southern African region have a very low rainfall. In these areas there is an increasing scarcity of water, which is particularly evident in the use of water as a result of the rapid population growth and urbanisation. It is thus important that governments should have strict control over the available water and that they should find options for saving water. Improved planning and an integrated approach to land and water management that involves the public sector and the communities is our only chance of survival.
- Poverty is closely related to continued high fertility rates, which eventually lead to rural and urban environmental degradation. Governments must be encouraged by the people of their countries to enhance the access of the rural and urban poor to employment opportunities, education, health and family planning. Community participation and the collaboration of all sectors and interest groups should be considered to improve the delivery of these services.
- Governments, the private sector and international organisations should find serious solutions for problems related to environmentally displaced persons. This includes the provision of support and assistance to areas most affected by this problem. A definite continuous programme should be implemented to eliminate the root causes of these problems.
- Areas that are highly vulnerable to natural disasters such as floods (e.g. KwaZulu-Natal) and veldfires (Eastern Cape) should be assisted in minimising the ensuing hazards to the environment and human health and safety. This may be achieved by planning land use and promoting emergency preventive measures and preparedness.
- International organisations are urged to increase their assistance in the form of sharing technology, training, policy formulation and expertise on the integration of population and environment-related factors in national planning.
- Greater awareness should be created through the formal education system.
- Research should be undertaken to identify critically endangered areas beset by population pressures, pollution, destruction of the ecosystem and the degradation of resources.
- Special attention should be given to improving the plight of indigenous populations. Their culture should be protected, but their harmful practices should be discouraged.
- Conflicting goals should be negotiated and attainable goals and solutions should be created with mutual gains.

The role of the Primary Health Care Professional must not be underestimated. These professionals do not sit in sterile offices but are out there in the community where they work and live. They are in the homes, at work, school and in the heart of the community from which they themselves come. They have the influence and they are trusted – they can make a difference.

4.15 SUMMARY

It is clear from this chapter that the world is filling up with people at an alarming rate and that this is leading towards a universal tragedy. The role of the nurse must not be ignored or underestimated. Nurses, however, may only contribute if they are knowledgeable and if they actively participate in the communities they serve. This chapter is by no means a comprehensive text. The nurse remains a perpetual student. It is therefore her own responsibility to keep up to date.

QUESTIONS

1. Discuss the concepts of demography and population.
2. Define the following concepts:
   (a) demographic transition
   (b) mortality rate
   (c) fertility rate
   (d) migration
   (e) lifespan
   (f) life expectancy.
3. Discuss the global consequences of uncontrolled population growth.
4. Describe how the community nurse can participate in uplifting living standards for the people in the community with a high population growth.
5. Write short notes on why individuals reject contraception.
6. Describe the consequences of uncontrolled population growth in the South African population.

FURTHER READING

Marais, H.C. (ed.) 1988. *South Africa: perspectives on the future.* Pinetown: Owen Burgess.

Raubenheimer, P. 1987. *Demografiese patrone: die Suid-Afrikaanse situasie.* Stellenbosch: Universiteitsuitgewers- en Boekhandelaars.

South Africa. 1983. *Demographic trends in South Africa. A report of the Science Committee of the President's Council.* Johannesburg: Lex Patria.

BIBLIOGRAPHY

Central Statistical Services. 1994. *Population census.* Pretoria: Government Printer.

Chimere-Dan, O. 1993. *In search of explanations for fertility and reproductive behaviour in Africa.* Johannesburg: African Studies Institute.

Marais, H.C. (ed.) 1988. *South Africa: perspectives on the future.* Pinetown: Owen Burgess.

Mausner, J.S. & Bahn, A.K. 1974. *Epidemiology: an introductory text.* Philadelphia: W.B. Saunders.

Raubenheimer, P. 1987. *Demografiese patrone: die Suid-Afrikaanse situasie.* Stellenbosch: Universiteitsuitgewers- en Boekhandelaars.

University of Cape Town. 1994. *SALDRU Report.* Cape Town: UCT.

University of Cape Town. 1993. *DBSA for SALDRU.* Cape Town: UCT.

5 Epidemiology in community health care

SUSAN HATTINGH

CHAPTER OBJECTIVES

After reading this chapter, the student should be able to:

- define the term "epidemiology";
- define key concepts often used in epidemiology;
- describe the determinants of disease;
- write short notes on the aims and uses of epidemiology;
- distinguish between morbidity and mortality rates;
- identify the sources of data for epidemiological studies;
- discuss the epidemiological process; and
- describe the role of the nurse in epidemiology.

5.1 INTRODUCTION

Epidemiology has its roots in Biblical times and in the writings of the Greek physician Hippocrates. *The Aphorisms of Hippocrates* (fifth century B.C.) contain careful observations of a large number of case studies on diseases. In the publication *Airs, Waters, Places,* timeless advice on good environmental epidemiology is offered (in Last 1987:27):

> Whoever would study medicine aright must learn of the following subjects. First he must consider the effect of each of the seasons of the year and the differences between them. Secondly he must study the warm and the cold winds, both those which are common to every country and those peculiar to a particular locality. Lastly, the effect of water on the health must not be forgotten . . . When, therefore, a physician comes to a district previously unknown to him, he should consider both its situation and its aspect to the winds . . . Similarly, the nature of the water supply must be considered . . . Then think of the soil, whether it be bare and waterless or thickly covered with vegetation and well-watered; whether in a hollow and stifling, or exposed and cold. Lastly consider the life of the inhabitants themselves; are they heavy drinkers and eaters and consequently unable to stand fatigue or, being fond of work and exercise, eat wisely but drink sparely?

In ancient times this method was used to study epidemic diseases and, because of the lack of knowledge about intervention and the prevention of diseases, physicians could do little more than observe and record the mortality rate among sufferers. Until the Renaissance, physicians rarely recorded diseases and their observations were generalised and based on impressions rather than on empirical evidence. Subsequently, up to the Reformation, disease was attributed to harmful forces and was either thought to be the result of the intervention of harmful spirits, or a punishment for transgressions, or even a trial of faith.

Epidemiology made great strides with the introduction of statistics. John Grant was the first to describe the methods and the uses of numerical records in his publication *Natural and Political Observations on the Bill of Mortality* in 1662, and he is often regarded as the founder of vital statistics in epidemiology.

In the 19th century, epidemiologists developed a painstaking system of monitoring diseases. This system consisted of collecting and recording information based on careful clinical observation, precise counts of well-defined cases and demonstrations of relationships between cases and the characteristics of the population in which they occurred. Through the work of various researchers, specific diseases and specific agents were identified as causative elements in specific health problems. It is believed that John Snow, when visiting sufferers of cholera in 1854, investigated the companies that supplied the drinking water in London. He discovered that the people who contracted cholera got their water from the polluted part of the Thames, and that this water was supplied by a specific company. Through this epidemiological study, he collected facts about the disease, thus demonstrating the mode of transmission about 30 years before Koch isolated and identified the cholera *vibrio*.

William Farr (1807–1883) was another great scientist who contributed a great deal to the fields of vital statistics and epidemiology. He defined and clarified many basic concepts such as the scope of epidemiology, the relationship between mortality rates and the probability of dying, immunity, dose-response relationships, and the relationship between incidence and prevalence. He was also the first effectively to classify diseases.

In England alone, one fourth of the population died from the plague in the 14th century, and this trend continued in Europe for more than three centuries. It later spread to Japan and here a Japanese bacteriologist, Kitasato, discovered the plague bacillus after the disease had spread to Hong Kong. It was only after ten years that the web of causation of this disease was traced from rats to fleas to man.

Florence Nightingale (1820–1910) laid the foundations of epidemiology in nursing during the Crimean War. Forty out of every 100 British soldiers were dying in the Crimea before Florence Nightingale instituted environmental and nutritional changes in the hospitals and in the field. When her work was completed, the mortality rate had dropped to two per cent. The core concept of her writings is the importance of the environment. She viewed the environment as the external conditions that influence and affect life, and she emphasised the physical surroundings rather than the psychological or social environments. She stressed aspects such as ventilation, clean air, clean water, warmth and overall cleanliness, as seen in Figure 5.1. Miss Nightingale thus regarded the physical condition of the individual as dependent on the environment; patient and nature function together. She viewed the cleanliness of the physical environment as a direct factor in the prevention of disease and in the lowering of mortality rates. She also kept detailed records and careful descriptions of the health conditions in the Crimean military camps, and these are viewed as one of the first systematic descriptive studies of the distribution and patterns of disease in a population.

FIGURE 5.1: The physical environment as described by Florence Nightingale

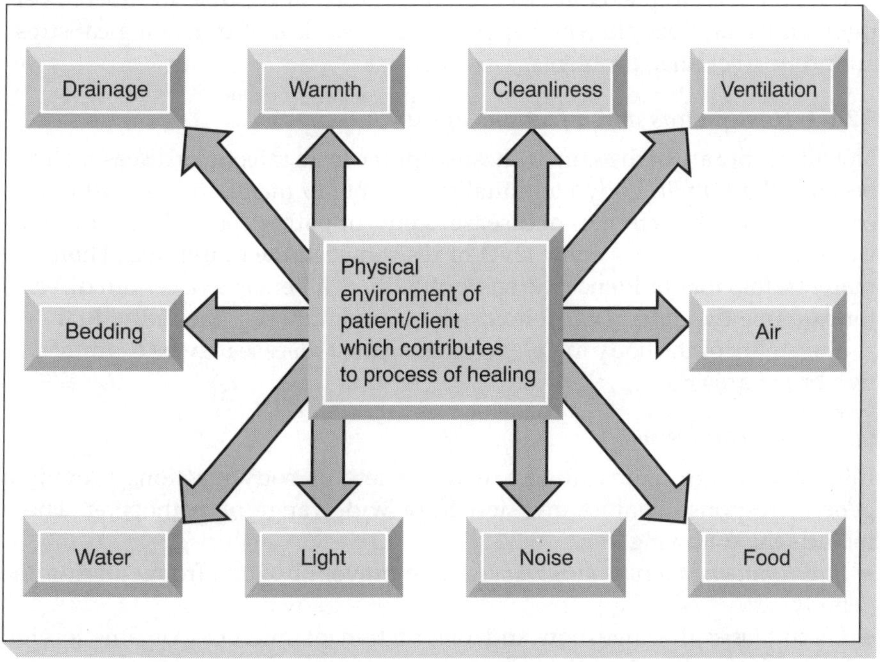

Through the decades further advances were made in epidemiology and it was during World War II that the pure emphasis on communicable diseases changed and risks associated with heart disease, lung cancer and other public health problems were identified and studied for the first time.

5.2 THE DETERMINANTS OF DISEASES

Although it has been stressed earlier that epidemiology is not only concerned with the study of diseases, but also with the study of other health-related phenomena, both communicable diseases and non-communicable diseases are present in communities and therefore need specific attention. Through studying the determinants of diseases, the factors that may cause illness can be isolated. The three broad factors that describe these determinants are the host (intrinsic), the environment (extrinsic) and the agent.

5.2.1 The host (intrinsic factors)

The forces in man and the forces in the environment in which he lives influence his state of health. From this point of view, man is the host to disease agents. Factors that will determine the susceptibility of the individual to a certain disease include age, sex, race, genetic make-up, immunological status, nutritional status, pregnancy, psychological status and previous diseases. For example, children are much more susceptible to tuberculosis than adults, and people who experience a great deal of psychological stress are prone to cardiac problems.

5.2.1.1 Host factors and infectious agents

Not all people are in the same way susceptible to an infectious disease. This is because the human body continually attempts to maintain homeostasis by counteracting the activities of disease agents or pathogens with specific antibodies, resulting in a specific level of resistance in the individual. There are many factors that influence the susceptibility of a person to a certain disease, for example the nutritional status, age or constitution of the individual.

The ability of the body to defend itself against disease may be examined in two broad areas:

(a) Non-specific resistance

Inherited factors representing a wide variety of body reactions provide a general response against invasion by a wide range of pathogens. These include the following:

- *Intact skin and mucous membranes:* these prevent bacteria from entering the body.
- *Phagocytosis:* the ingestion and destruction of microbes or any foreign particulate matter by cells called phagocytes.
- *Inflammation:* when cells are damaged by microbes, physical agents or chemical agents, the injury sets off an inflammatory reaction or response and the injury is viewed as a form of stress. Inflammation is thus a defence mechanism of the body against stress due to tissue damage.
- *Fever:* an abnormally high body temperature which is caused most frequently by infection from bacteria and their toxins as well as by viruses. A high body temperature inhibits some microbic growth and speeds up reactions that aid repair.
- *Antimicrobic substances:* these are produced by the body to ward off infectious agents. These include interferon, complement and properdin.

(b) Specific resistance

Immunity or specific resistance involves the production of a specific antibody or specific cell against a specific pathogen or its toxin. The components of specific resistance include the following:

- *Antigens:* any chemical substance that causes the body to produce specific antibodies and/or specific cells called T-cells, which react with the antigen.
- *Antibodies:* a protein produced by the body in response to the presence of an antigen, which is capable of combining specifically with the antigen and which could be naturally acquired when a person recovered from that specific disease, or artificially, e.g. when antigens are artificially introduced to the body through immunisation.
- *Cellular and humeral immunity:* the ability of the body to defend itself against invading agents such as bacteria, toxins, viruses and foreign tissues. Cellular immunity is the formation of specialised sensitised lymphocytes by the body that have the ability to attach themselves to the foreign agent and to destroy it. Humeral immunity is the formation of circulating antibodies that are capable of attacking an invading agent.

5.2.1.2 *Host factors that lead to the development of a disease*

A person who is affected by a disease may either be well or ill, depending on a variety of factors. The factors that influence the development of the disease include:

- *The amount of the agent to which the host is exposed:* this will determine the probability of the host becoming ill. For example, if a person takes a moderate amount of alcohol, he or she will normally not become ill, but excessive intake of alcohol may cause serious illness. The same principle applies to the infectious agent to which the host is exposed. If a host has limited exposure to *Mycobacterium tuberculosis* and his nutritional and general physical status is good, he will most likely not develop the disease. However, the more the host is exposed to micro-organisms or any other disease agents, the higher the risk of infection or disease.
- *The general physical state of the individual:* someone in good health, who exercises regularly, rests and sleeps well, eats a balanced meal every day, and lives a healthy, moderate life-style, when exposed to severe stress, may resist heart disease and ulcers better than someone in poorer general health.
- *The pathogenicity of the agent:* this describes the tendency of the agent concerned to cause an adverse reaction in the person.
- *The virulence of the agent:* this denotes the malignancy of the specific agent to which the person has been exposed.

There are, however, many unanswered questions about the role of host factors and disease. We do not know, for example, why certain very heavy smokers do not develop lung cancer.

5.2.1.3 *Genetic factors*

There are a number of genetic factors that have been identified as relating either to an increased or decreased susceptibility to certain diseases. For example, a deficiency of one specific enzyme, alpha-1-antitrypsin, is associated with a type of chronic obstructive lung disease, and sickle-cell anaemia is associated with a decreased risk of malaria due to the presence of *Plasmodium falciparum*.

5.2.1.4 *Personality factors*

It is well known that there is a relationship between personality and disease. Personality variables do influence the course of illness. For example, some people, due to personality traits, refuse to seek medical care in due time, or do not adhere to treatment prescribed to them. Also, there is a definite relationship between coronary heart disease and personality traits. The rates for coronary heart disease are higher in people characterised by aggression, competitiveness, ambition, restlessness and a sense of time urgency. However, one particular factor alone is not sufficient to account for a disease or/ and condition. A sequence of events usually leads up to a disease or condition.

5.2.1.5 *Social class*

Social class membership is a host attribute which contributes to disease. Developmental experiences and life-style are intimately tied to one's state of health and some diseases show a differential frequency among persons of different social classes.

5.2.2 Environmental factors (extrinsic)

The term "environment" refers to all external or extrinsic conditions and influences life. This is the aspect of community health that is concerned with all the factors, circumstances and conditions in the environment surrounding the patient that may exert an influence on his or her health and well-being, either physically or mentally, whether in the work-place, the home or the social sphere.

The environmental factors that determine the host's exposure to a specific agent may include:

- living conditions;
- overcrowding;
- hygienic conditions;
- environmental conditions such as the state of roads, traffic and lighting;
- occupation;
- climatic and seasonal changes;
- geographical location;
- pollution; and
- the life-style of the individual.

Environmental factors thus include all the living conditions (even before birth) and it has been found that there are significant associations between determinants and diseases. By examining the characteristics of people and places and by taking into account the time of year, on comparing them with diseases, one can narrow down the suspected agents of the diseases concerned.

Disease cannot be attributed to any one factor alone. Host and environment both play an important role in producing a disease. By recognising this interrelationship and understanding the cause(s) of the disease, one may discover clues to primary prevention and preventative strategies can then be worked out.

The environment in which a human being function forms part of an integrated eco-system. Many environmental aspects are also interrelated, but in an attempt to understand diseases caused by the environment, a broad classification of biological, physical and social environment is often used:

5.2.2.1 *The biological environment*

The biological environment encompasses the following:

- the infectious agents of the disease, e.g. virus, bacteria;
- reservoirs of infection - this includes other human beings, animals and soil;
- vectors that may transmit diseases such as a fleas, mosquitoes and lice; and
- plants and animals, e.g. tobacco, plants and animals as sources of food.

5.2.2.2 *The socio-economic environment*

The socio-economic environment is the overall economic and political organisation of a society and of the institutions by which individuals and groups are integrated into that society at various stages of their lives. There are many social and economic aspects to the life of an individual that affect his or her health.

Diseases are spread under certain specific conditions that may be related to the economic status of a community, such as:

- housing;
- sanitation;
- water supply;
- food hygiene;
- disposal of refuse; and
- the availability and acceptability of health services.

The socio-economic status of a group may also contribute to psychological stress. Many social problems such as suicide and child abuse are associated with a poor socio-economic climate in a community. Those who are the poorest also tend to be the least healthy and the consequences of poverty, such as poor nutrition, unsatisfactory living conditions and inadequate education, medical services and stimulation, tend to lead to high physical and psychological disease rates.

Particular social customs and cultural practices may further affect health. The types of foods eaten, childbearing practices and traditional medicines, customs and beliefs may all influence the disease patterns in a community. Another important aspect of the social environment is the general level of receptivity to new ideas in the community. Resistance to new ideas may develop if deeply held practices and beliefs are violated.

Economic development frequently results in industrialisation and urbanisation. The consequences are the disruption of cultures, the weakening of family ties and the creation of communities where support for the less competent members (such as vagrants, the unemployed and abusers of alcohol and drugs) has to be provided by social welfare services rather than by integrated communities.

5.2.2.3 *The physical environment*

The physical environment includes all physical aspects such as heat, light, air, water, radiation, gravity, atmospheric pressure and chemical agents. We have much control over our physical environment through the provision of adequate shelter, the use of water supplies, the treatment of sewage and the use and misuse of fauna and flora. With rapid population growth, our physical environment has become the focus of serious attention, and problems such as the increase in pollution from vehicles, industrial wastes and noise require active intervention.

The weather, climate and seasonal changes are important indicators of disease in the environment, as are the topography and geography of a particular area. Climate not only regulates the fauna and flora of an area, but it also has an influence on parasites and their survival and transmission. For example, salmonella found in contaminated food, multiplies in a warm, humid climate, and the Anopheles mosquito, which transmits malaria, thrives in warm, tropical areas of a country.

5.2.3 The agent

The agent must be thought of as a substance, living or inanimate, or a force, the presence or absence of which is the "cause" of the disease or condition. The agent may be described as a factor, the presence or absence of which causes a disease. When a factor must be present for a disease to occur, it is called an agent of that disease. For example, the influenza virus is the agent of influenza.

Agents may come from any sphere of the environment as described above and may be classified as:

- *Biological:* insects, worms, fungi, bacteria, rickettsia, metazoa, protozoa and viruses that cause infectious diseases.

- *Physical:* mechanical forces that may cause accidents or injuries and abnormalities in the atmosphere (extreme temperatures, radioactivity, lead, asbestos)
- *Chemical:* dusts, gases, vapours, fumes, liquids (acids, alkalis), poisons, allergens
- *Genetic:* the transmission of diseases from parent to child through genes (Huntington's chorea, trisomy 21)
- *Psychological:* any stressful circumstances in the environment under which a person may live
- *Nutritional:* excesses or deficiencies of the basic nutritional components necessary to maintain life (proteins, vitamins, minerals).

5.3 DEFINING EPIDEMIOLOGY

It can be said that the science of epidemiology has its origins in the investigation of outbreaks of infectious diseases. In contemporary health sciences, however, the scope of epidemiology and its applications have been greatly extended and include all health-related phenomena such as suicide, divorce, motor vehicle accidents, child abuse, genetic disorders, chronic conditions such as cancer or Alzheimer's disease and many more.

There are many and varied definitions of epidemiology. The word "epidemiology" is derived from the Greek words *epi, demos* and *logos* which, literally translated, mean "science of the people". The word also reminds us that the first concern of epidemiologists is to investigate and control epidemics.

According to Last (1987:31), epidemiology is the study of the distribution and determinants of health-related events in defined populations, and the application of this study to the control of health problems.

Stanhope and Lancaster (1996:912–16) describe epidemiology as the study of the determination of health status and of the determinants of deviations from health in populations.

Clark (1984:131) describes epidemiology as the study of the factors that influence the incidence, distribution and control of disease, defect, disability and death.

Epidemiology is seen as a study that explains the aetiology of specific injuries and diseases, identifies and describes factors that contribute to health or illness, and provides the basis for developing and evaluating community health programmes to promote health and to prevent disease.

From the definitions it becomes clear that epidemiology is concerned with the extent and types of illnesses, whether physical, mental or social, that occur in groups of people, and with the factors that influence the distribution of these illnesses. It is furthermore important to realise that the distribution of all health-related phenomena is related to time (e.g. a specific season, night or day, specific hours such as peak traffic hours), place (a specific geographic area, a specific country, a specific workplace, etc.) and person (groups of individuals in a specific age group, of a specific gender, of a specific occupation, of a specific culture, etc). Different health issues present themselves differently in different communities and groups of people.

The results of epidemiological studies are therefore essential for planning, prioritising and evaluating health services. Epidemiology is practised within a team and members such as health planners, statisticians, doctors, nurses, dentists, veterinarians, health authorities or funders from private sectors and even members of communities and groups within communities are involved in collecting, collating, analysing and evaluating data. Because community nurses are actively involved in and with groups and communities, they form valuable members of the epidemiological team. The community nurse's involvement is depicted in Figure 5.2.

5.4 THE VALUE AND USE OF EPIDEMIOLOGICAL STUDIES

Epidemiologists strive to attain answers to the following questions:

- What is the incidence of diseases in a community?
- Is there an increase or a decrease in health status of a particular group over time?
- Does one geographical area have a higher frequency of a specific disease than another geographical area?
- Do certain people have special characteristics that are related to certain diseases?
- Why do some people recover more quickly than others from a particular disease?
- Is one kind of treatment superior to another and, if so, why?

Note the relationship to time, place and person in these questions.

Epidemiological studies address the cause(s) of disease; the distribution of the disease in people in relation to age, sex, race, occupation and social characteristics; exposure to certain specific agents; susceptibility to diseases; the influence of the environment on health; genetic determinants or other characteristics that are prominent in a certain individual or group. Disease-related attributes and contributory factors to disease are also studied by using the epidemiological method. Aspects such as the use of tobacco, alcohol, attitudes towards life and disease, stress and numerous other factors also have an influence on health-related phenomena.

With the wealth of information available from epidemiologic studies:

- specific existing and/or new health needs within specific communities or groups can be identified;
- the cause, determinants, contributing factors and distribution of health-related issues can be described;

FIGURE 5.2: The involvement of the community nurse in epidemiology

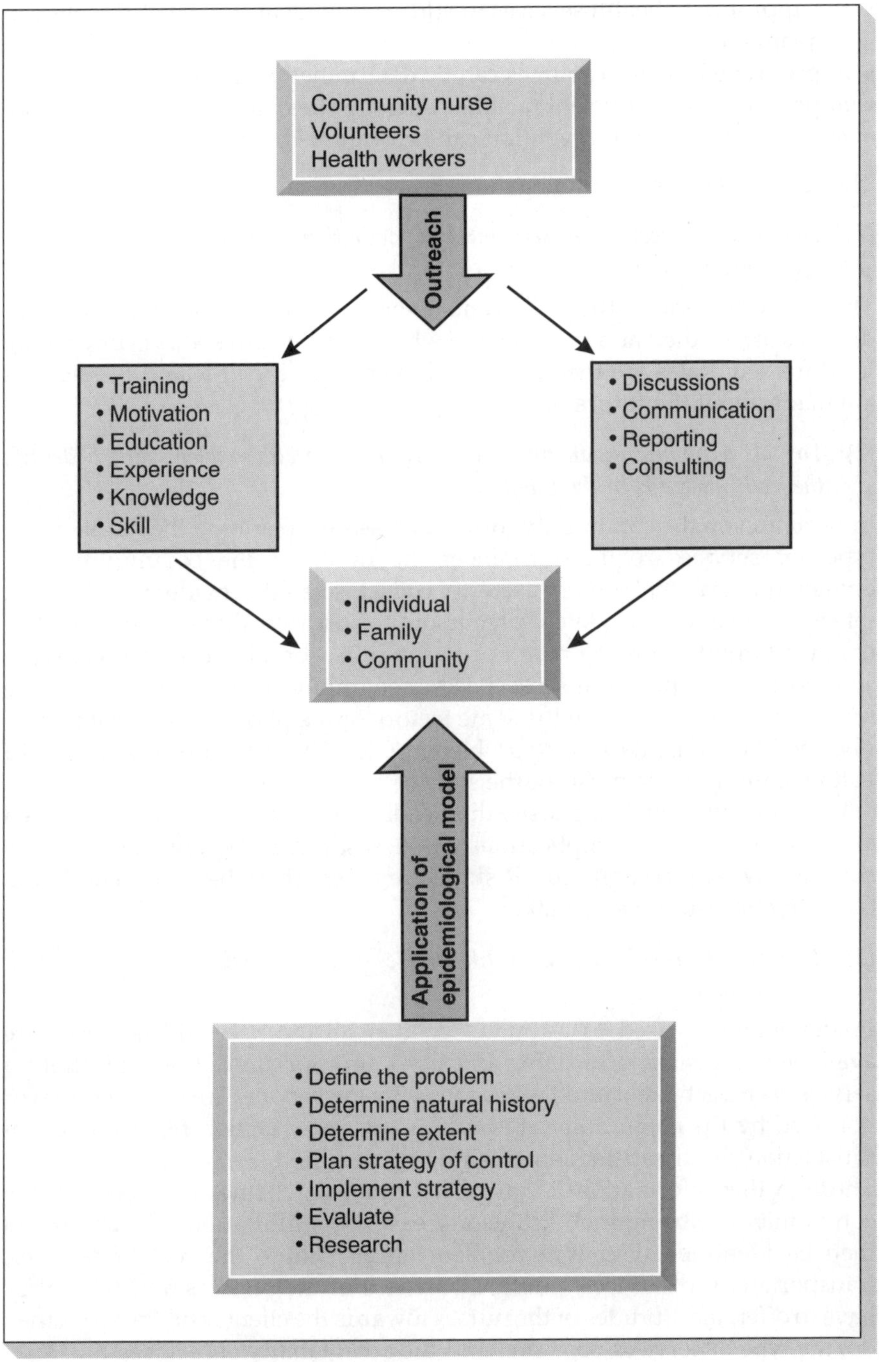

- health needs can be prioritised;
- the appropriate health services to address the identified health issues can be planned;
- appropriate human resources can be determined and trained;
- appropriate and sufficient facilities and supplies can be determined; and
- the effect of health intervention can be evaluated and adapted.

The seven uses of epidemiology are:

(1) *To study the effects of disease states in populations over a time and to predict future health needs*

This is the historical study of events over a specific period. The trends of diseases are studied and the question whether the health status is improving is addressed. Rates are then compared over a specific time and predictions are made about the future of specific groups.

(2) *To make a community diagnosis to determine the health problems and to identify the health hazards in the community*

Information on the community forms the basis for planning the number and types of services required to meet the needs of the community. The epidemiological method is used to collect scientific evidence of death, infection, diseases, accidents, precursors to diseases, disasters or threat of disaster. Groups with common needs, interests, complaints or problems are studied, for example groups in a specific geographical area, children from the same school, workers from the same factory or members of the same family. The needs, complaints and/or problems of the risk group are analysed and a valid community diagnosis of the state of health is made.

With a community diagnosis, the needs of the population are identified and the burden and implications of diseases already prevailing in the community are recognised. Risk factors can then be eliminated and corrective measures can be taken.

(3) *To evaluate the efficiency of health services and the effectiveness of health programmes*

Epidemiology is used to estimate whether all the necessary services are available, accessible, affordable and used appropriately. The utilisation of services is investigated and the reasons why the services are either chosen or not used by the community are investigated. Information regarding client satisfaction or dissatisfaction is gathered routinely or by special survey. Through this information it can be determined whether the needs of the community are being met. Problem areas in the utilisation of services can then be identified. Potential problem areas include the cost of services, transportation to services, public awareness of the services and what they have to offer, the attitudes of the nurses towards the clients and the work they do, the type of services provided and the acceptability of services.

The data collected serve as a monitoring device and are useful in the evaluation of the services provided. By keeping a close watch on mortality and morbidity rates, the effectiveness of the service can be determined.

(4) *To estimate individual risk from group experience*

Risk refers to the probability of developing an unfavourable disease, condition or illness. Epidemiological methods are used to collect the appropriate data and to estimate the likelihood that people who are exposed to the risk factors of a particular disease will contract it. It is also possible to determine whether there is a likelihood of developing a disease at a later stage.

To reduce the chances of future disease or injury, the possible harmful consequences of certain factors or behaviours are identified by the epidemiologist and an attempt is made clearly to delineate and quantify these factors. The objective is to describe illness or injury in populations in terms of risk factors so that the appropriate intervention may be planned to reduce risks in the community, thus to prevent and control disease.

Risk factors may be influenced by a patient's individual characteristics, such as age, sex and genetic make-up, or factors in the internal or external environment that are potentially alterable. It is inherited risk that determines the probability of getting cancer, diabetes or any other disease or condition. Families at risk of cystic fibrosis may provide excellent information for estimating the risk for future genetic transmission of this disease. These cases are carefully recorded and a surveillance system is developed to educate the public.

It is our life-style in the environment in which we live that determines the risk factors to which we are exposed. This principle may be illustrated in various ways, for example, accidents are a major risk of life and if alcohol is taken before driving, this risk will become even greater. Also, it is well known that obesity and an inactive life-style contribute to heart disease, and workers in industries that make use of substances such as lead, asbestos and radioactive material are at risk of developing serious diseases. By identifying these risk factors, health programmes can be instituted to change high risk behaviours such as overeating and/or smoking.

Epidemiology is therefore used to identify risks for the individual and the group. Information is collected from ongoing observation of any hazardous event that may cause disease, accident or death. To prevent accidents, injury or disease, one must be able to identify the causes and the means by which disease agents are transmitted and eradicated.

However, in the identification of risks, careful observation, monitoring and recording are essential. Through the identification of risks, and through the education and guidance of clients, corrective measures can be taken. For example, in industry injuries or diseases such as asbestosis can be prevented.

(5) *To identify syndromes*

Disease classification and the identification of syndromes are directly related to clinical medicine. Signs and symptoms thought to be similar can be collected through the use of the epidemiological method. Investigation sometimes makes it possible to group together certain differing manifestations of a condition or to separate identical diseases into more than one category. For instance, gonorrhoea and syphilis were once regarded as the same disease. However, through their epidemiological characteristics such as incubation periods, two different organisms were identified. The distinction between Hepatitis A and Hepatitis B is also an example of the identification of differing signs and symptoms through the use of epidemiology. Tuberculosis, measles, AIDS and many other diseases have distinct manifestations that distinguish them from one another.

(6) *To complete the clinical picture of a particular problem*

One of the most important uses of epidemiology is the completion of the clinical picture or natural development of the disease before the disease becomes irreversible. Preventative intervention is possible in most instances if accurate identification and diagnosis take place.

The early recognition, diagnosis, and timeous and effective treatment to prevent complications, chronicity and/or spread of diseases require an understanding and a knowledge of the disease as well as the identification of the high risk groups. Malaria, as an example, is a disease that is geographically determined. By also knowing that the precursor is the Anopheles mosquito, which breeds in low-lying marshes, and that the high-risk groups are those people living in the geographical areas where the mosquito is found, malaria can be prevented or limited by controlling stagnant water, spraying low-lying marshes and taking precautions not to be bitten by the mosquito.

The risk of cardiovascular disease can be detected before the actual disease is identified or diagnosed because of the known facts that high cholesterol and lipid levels, high blood pressure and psychological stress are contributing factors to the disease. By controlling these precursors, the risk of getting the disease is diminished. The detection of precursors is possible through screening populations, identifying high risk groups and through delivering services to control the precursors rather than the disease. For example, the mortality rate in diabetics can be limited if the precursors of complications can be eliminated. By adopting a healthy diet and life-style, the complications of the disease can be limited.

(7) *To search for the causes of disease*

This is the most obvious use of epidemiology. When the cause of a disease, illness or condition is known, such as smallpox, measles, polio and whooping cough, preventative measures, e.g. immunisation, can be introduced to control the disease. The causative agents of these diseases were determined through epidemiologic observations and analysis.

In the case of HIV/AIDS, accurate and analytical epidemiological studies made the isolation of the virus and the description of the disease process possible. Only with this knowledge, can attempts be made to find ways to prevent the spread of the disease.

5.5 MODELS USED IN EPIDEMIOLOGY

Models are often designed to guide and explain actions and/or activities. Models in epidemiology developed and changed in accordance with the developments and changes that occurred in the discipline itself.

5.5.1 The epidemiological triad

This model was developed by Lilienfeld to explain a disease in terms of the relationship and interaction between the susceptible host, the causative agent and the environment within which this interaction occurs. This triad is depicted in Figure 5.3. A change in any of the components will alter an existing equilibrium to increase or decrease the frequency of disease. This particular model was used when the emphasis of epidemiological studies was on communicable diseases and, in particular, infectious diseases.

5.5.2 The epidemiological dyad

The epidemiological dyad, consisting of only two components, namely the host and the environment, was developed when not only bacterial diseases, but also diseases with a causative agent in a physico-chemical, socio-economic or genetic environment were studied. In this model the causative agent is regarded as an integral and therefore inseparable part of the environment. This model is depicted in Figure 5.4.

5.5.3 The chain of causation

The chain of causation was developed by epidemiologists to describe the sequence of events that takes place when a disease occurs. The chain begins with a reservoir, which is a safe place for an agent to live and multiply. For example, bacteria may live and multiply within man. This agent must, however, have a portal of exit and a mode of transmission or a portal of entry into the host.

5.5.4 The web of causation

This is a more recent model used to describe the cause of diseases. This model was put forward by MacMahon and his colleagues in 1960. The web of

FIGURE 5.3: The epidemiological triad model

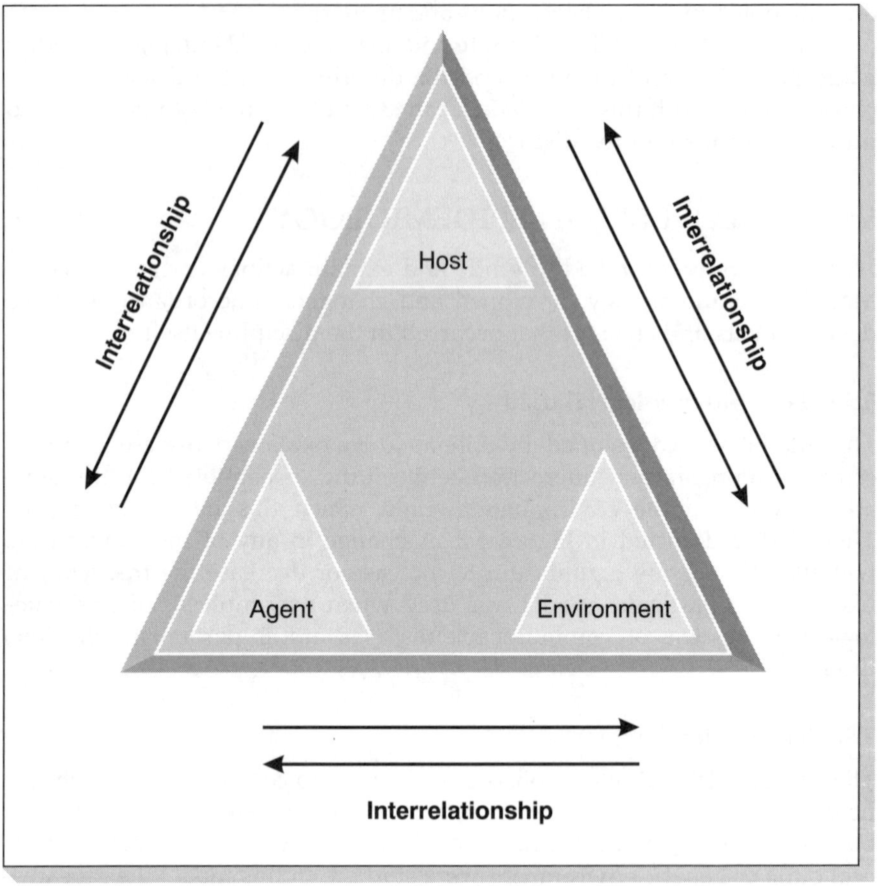

FIGURE 5.4: The epidemiological dyad model

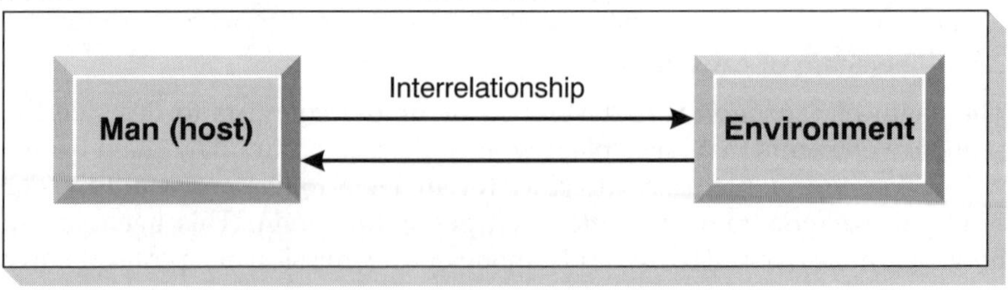

causation is an advanced concept that explains the intricacies and multiple nature of factors and events in the development of disease. This concept also serves as a guideline for applying preventative measures in epidemiological practice.

FIGURE 5.5: Chain of causation in infectious disease

Example: Malaria

Reservoir:	Human/primates
Portal of exit:	Bite of *Anopheles* mosquito from infected person
Mode of transmission:	Blood of infected person
Agent:	*Plasmodium falciparum*
Portal of entry:	Bite of *Anopheles* mosquito
Host:	Human/primates

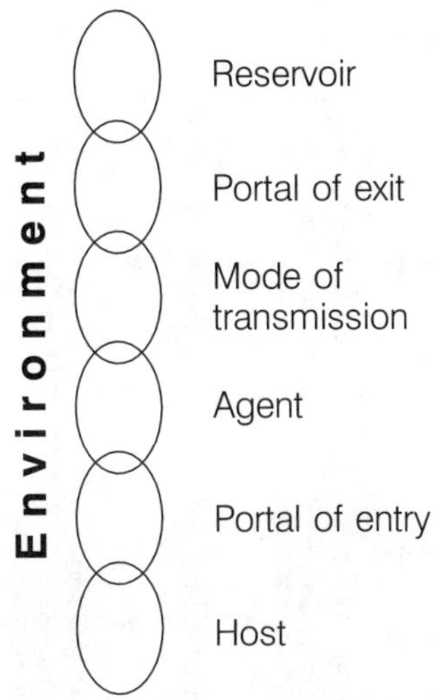

Figure 5.6 explains the web of causation of the various interrelated factors that cause malnutrition, and interventions for its prevention and the promotion of health are indicated.

5.6 THE CLASSIFICATION OF EPIDEMIOLOGICAL STUDIES

Epidemiological studies can be classified in various ways. The purpose of some sort of classification is to organise or group together a number of similar issues, events, activities or objects to enhance clarity, understanding and utilisation. In this particular classification, epidemiological studies are divided into two broad categories.

5.6.1 Descriptive or observational studies

These studies are concerned with the observation of the distribution and progression of a disease in a particular community or population and the description thereof. Taking the time of the events that are studied as the distinguishing characteristic, descriptive studies can be further subdivided.

5.6.1.1 Case-control studies

These describe a retrospective "flash-back" of a particular event, disease, disease pattern or any health-related phenomenon. This health-related event,

FIGURE 5.6: Multiple causation of nutritional problems

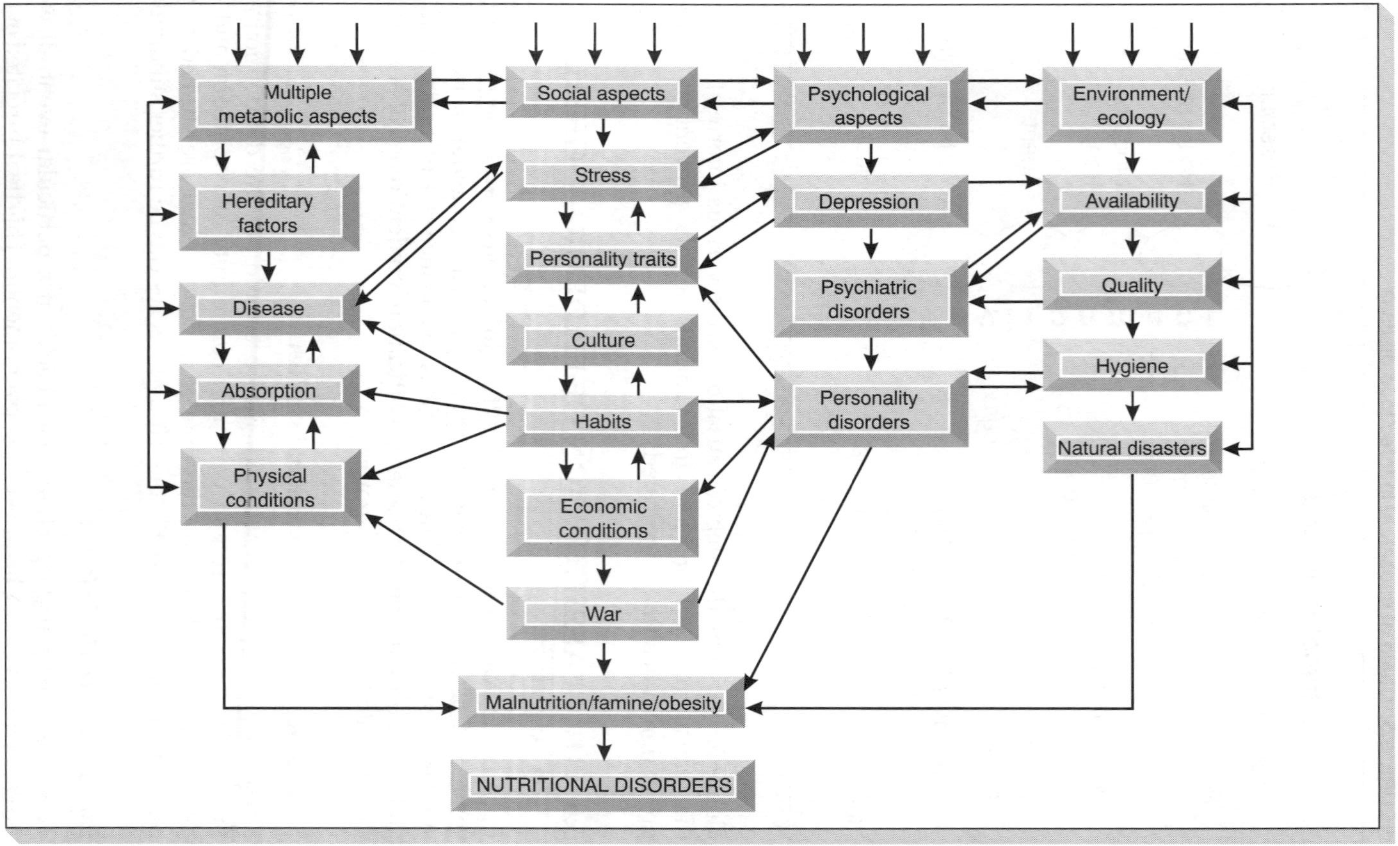

which has already occurred, is analysed and described in such a way that it is better understood, in an attempt to derive information and knowledge from the study that could be utilised in the future prevention and/or control of a similar health phenomenon.

5.6.1.2 *Health-related survey studies*

These describe a "snap-shot" of existing or current health situations. The information collected from surveys is often used to determine the existing health status of a particular group or community. Disease-causing agents and contributing factors could be determined through surveys and the information used to prevent or control a health-related phenomenon. Surveys are also effective in evaluating the impact of health interventions on the attitudes, perceptions, knowledge, values or health behaviour in groups or populations.

5.6.1.3 *Cohort studies*

These focus on a "newsreel of events". These studies are continuous in nature. They start at a particular time in a particular study population and continue on that same aspect in the same study population into the future. These studies are used to determine the changes that occur in populations over time and identify reasons for the changes and relationships between contributing factors, events and variables.

5.6.2 Experimental studies

Experimental studies in epidemiology are concerned with measuring any effects of the environment that are thought to be harmful, by applying control programmes to prevent, cure and rehabilitate the community or population. Experimental studies on human beings (and other living organisms) are often controversial and involve many ethical decisions. Experimental studies in the form of control-clinical trials are the most common form of experimental study in epidemiology.

5.7 THE EPIDEMIOLOGIC METHOD

Epidemiology is a scientific discipline. The method used to conduct an epidemiologic study therefore strongly resembles any acceptable scientific research method. The steps usually followed are illustrated in Table 5.1. It is important to note the following:

- Any epidemiologic study is limited and in many cases determined by the time and money available to complete the study.
- The literature study in an epidemiologic study cannot be listed as a particular consecutive step in the process or method. The reason for this is that available literature will be consulted on a continuous basis during all the steps of the epidemiologic method.

TABLE 5.1: The steps taken in an epidemiological study	
Steps	**Comments and clarification**
Describe the problem	• The problem observed should be clearly defined in terms of nature and extent
Determine the purpose of the study	• The purpose of the study should be clear. • In some instances epidemiologic studies can involve a big population and/or many aspects within a given population can be studied simultaneously.
Method	• The method will be determined by the purpose of the study, the nature of the information collected, the time available, and the money available • The method that is the most financially viable should be decided upon without losing sight of the purpose of the study • The variables that will influence the study must be identified and worked into the method • A method that will retain objectivity, credibility and reliability must be used.
Consent	• Informed consent for the study must be obtained from the appropriate authorities, groups and individuals.
Inputs	• The necessary input for effectively conducting the study should be determined, i.e. manpower, facilities, equipment and supplies.
Finances	• Application for financial support and/or sponsorship should be obtained. Full details of the study: the problem, value of the study, methods and target group, inputs as well as a specified budget should accompany the request for financial support.
Logistics	• The logistics should be prepared and finalised, eg forms printed, fieldworkers trained, accommodation and transport planned, procedure standardised. • All team members such as statisticians should be involved.
Pilot study	• A pilot study should be conducted on a small sample of the study population to determine and rectify any problems.
Collection and collation of data	• Standardised procedures should be followed. • Experts should be involved in the collation and interpretation of data if necessary.
Recommendations	• Make recommendations as early in the study as possible to enable decision makers to start intervention if necessary.
Feedback to periphery	• Feedback of the outcome of the study should be given to all role players at the periphery as a token of goodwill and appreciation.
Final report	• The final report should be finalised. • All team members should be acknowledged.

- Because epidemiologic studies often involve a team approach and because individuals and/or groups and communities are often utilised as sources from which data is collected, it is important, in addition to reporting the findings of an epidemiologic study in a scientific report, also to give practical and useful feedback on the findings to the team members and the individuals and groups involved in the study.

5.8 BASIC EPIDEMIOLOGICAL MEASUREMENTS

As pointed out in the definition of epidemiology, there is a necessity to measure or quantify diseases, accidents or conditions in various subgroups in the population or community. This measurement is done by relating cases to a population base. The fundamental concepts used in epidemiological measurements are counts, rates, incidence and prevalence.

Counts are the most simple and most frequently performed quantitative measurement used in epidemiology. A count is the number of persons in the group studied who have a particular disease or a particular characteristic. For example, it may be noted that children in a school hostel develop an infectious disease such as measles or that 28 women with cervical carcinoma come from rural areas.

Epidemiologists often base their statements on rates in which the numerator is the number of people with the disease or health-related phenomenon and the denominator is the population or the population at risk. This population (or the population at risk) must be in the same area at the same time. Rates are regarded as the only valid basis for comparisons.

It is one of the central concerns of epidemiology to find and enumerate appropriate denominators to describe and compare groups in a community in a meaningful and useful way. Vital statistics such as births, deaths and marriages are calculated as rates and form the basis of some of the most comprehensive data.

5.8.1 Morbidity rates

The prevalence and incidence rates are important indicators of morbidity (disease occurrence) in a specific population:

- The prevalence rate refers to the total number of existing cases of a disease or condition at a specific time. The prevalence rate is calculated on the basis of a particular period (t) and is reported in terms of the rate per 1 000 of the population.
- The incidence rate refers to the number of new cases of a particular disease or condition during a specific period.

The mortality and morbidity rates are extremely important to the epidemiologist. The mortality rate refers to the number of deaths as a result of a disease, whereas the morbidity rate reflects the occurrence of a specific health problem in the community that may or may not result in death. For example, the number of people who are affected by tuberculosis are referred to as the morbidity rate, but the number of people who die as a result of tuberculosis give the mortality rate.

5.8.2 Mortality rates

The overall mortality rate of a population (also referred to as the crude mortality rate) is calculated as follows:

TABLE 5.2: Important vital statistical rates	
Table type	**Population factor**
1 Rate	
Rate =	$\frac{\text{number of events (deaths, diseases, accidents) in a specific time period (t)*}}{\text{population in the same area (country, district, town), in the same specific time period (t)*}} \times \frac{1\,000}{1}$
2 Morbidity	
Prevalence rate =	$\frac{\text{number of cases with a disease (t)*}}{\text{total number in group (t)*}} \times \frac{1\,000}{1}$
Incidence rate =	$\frac{\text{number of new cases with a disease (t)*}}{\text{total population (t)*}} \times \frac{1\,000}{1}$
3 Mortality	
Crude mortality rate =	$\frac{\text{total number of deaths (t)*}}{\text{total population}} \times \frac{1\,000}{1}$
Age specific rate =	$\frac{\text{number of deaths at a particular age (t)*}}{\text{total number in same age group (t)*}} \times \frac{1\,000}{1}$
Case fatality rate =	$\frac{\text{number of deaths due to specific disease or cause (t)*}}{\text{total number with disease}} \times \frac{1\,000}{1}$
Maternal mortality rate =	$\frac{\text{number of deaths from puerperal causes during (t)*}}{\text{number of live births (t)*}} \times \frac{1\,000}{1}$
Infant mortality rate =	$\frac{\text{number of deaths at birth before age of 1 year (t)*}}{\text{number of live births (t)*}} \times \frac{1\,000}{1}$
Neonatal mortality rate =	$\frac{\text{number of deaths from birth to 28 days of age}}{\text{number of live births (t)*}} \times \frac{1\,000}{1}$
Foetal mortality rate =	$\frac{\text{number of foetal deaths between 20–28 weeks of gestation (t)*}}{\text{number of live births and foetal deaths}} \times \frac{1\,000}{1}$
Perinatal mortality rate =	$\frac{\text{number of perinatal deaths between 28 weeks of gestation to 1 week of age}}{\text{number of live births and foetal deaths at 28 weeks or more in same time}} \times \frac{1\,000}{1}$
* (t) = indicates a specific time period e.g. 1 year, 1 month or 1 week.	

$$\text{Crude mortality rate} = \frac{\text{total number of deaths/t}}{\text{total population/t}} \times \frac{1\,000}{1}$$

The mortality rate of any subgroup in a population can also be determined, for example an age-specific mortality rate.

$$\text{Age-specific mortality rate} = \frac{\text{number of deaths in a particular age group/t}}{\text{total number in same age group/t}} \times \frac{1\,000}{1}$$

Case fatality, or the cause-specific rate, refers to the number of people who die of a particular disease or cause. The time element may or may not be specified.

$$\text{Case fatality rate} = \frac{\text{number of deaths due to specific disease or cause/t}}{\text{total number with disease/t}} \times \frac{1\,000}{1}$$

The maternal mortality rate is usually determined over a period of one year and the denominator is the total of live births in that same year. It is calculated as follows:

$$\text{Maternal mortality rate} = \frac{\text{number of deaths from puerperal causes during/t}}{\text{number of live births/t}} \times \frac{1\,000}{1}$$

Various other rates, such as infant mortality, neonatal mortality, foetal mortality and perinatal mortality, are of significance to the community nurse and are calculated as follows:

$$\text{Infant mortality rate} = \frac{\text{number of deaths at birth or before the age of one year/t}}{\text{number of live births/t}} \times \frac{1\,000}{x}$$

$$\text{Neonatal mortality rate} = \frac{\text{number of deaths from birth to 28 days of age/t}}{\text{live births in same year}} \times \frac{1\,000}{1}$$

$$\text{Foetal mortality rate} = \frac{\text{number of foetal deaths between 20–28 weeks of gestation}}{\text{number of live births + foetal deaths}} \times \frac{1\,000}{1}$$

$$\text{Perinatal mortality rate} = \frac{\text{number of perinatal deaths between 28 weeks of gestation to 1 week of age}}{\text{number of live births + foetal deaths}} \times \frac{1\,000}{1}$$

Community nurses should utilise these rates to determine the health status of a particular community and to compare it with national or other applicable rates. Health statistics were not always accurately kept, were often not optimally utilised and were often inapplicable and insensitive to specific local health planning and evaluation. The Directorate Health Systems Research of the Department of Health is currently responsible for disease surveillance in South Africa. Statistics of all notifiable diseases as well as the reported AIDS cases are analysed and published on a monthly basis. This directorate is also responsible for developing an accessible and available health information system on a national basis. Collaboration, standardisation and coordination of all sectors related to health will be essential to attain a user-friendly and cost-effective health-information network.

All members of the health team should be involved in keeping accurate health statistics, collating them and using them on a daily, weekly, monthly and annual basis to monitor the health status of groups and communities, to identify new health trends and health needs and to evaluate the cost-effectiveness and quality of health-intervention strategies. The individual, social and economic value of informed and enabled healthy individuals and communities, the current cost of health facilities, supplies, equipment and health personnel are driving forces behind the urgency to plan, implement and evaluate according to objective, scientific, quantifiable and comparable criteria rather than to base health services on perceptions, feelings and political gain.

5.9 SOURCES OF DATA FOR EPIDEMIOLOGICAL STUDIES

There are some major sources of data from existing records, informal investigation and scientific studies, all of which are needed for the monitoring of health status and are used for epidemiological studies.

5.9.1 Existing data

5.9.1.1 Census data

Census data, which are usually updated once a decade (because of the cost and logistics involved), are perhaps the most important national source of data about total populations. Census data provide information on the numbers of persons and their demographic, socio-economic and household characteristics. This also provides the denominator of national morbidity and mortality statistics.

The term "census" comes from the Latin word meaning "to estimate or assess", and refers to periodic counts or enumerations of the population. The importance of these accurate counts is recognised by governments all over the world. This information is gathered to assist in the social and fiscal planning of a country.

Through census, many population characteristics necessary for epidemiological studies are identified, such as distribution in terms of geographical location, age, sex, race, marital status, religion, relation to the head of the household, occupation and income. Information from a census is vitally important because it forms the basis for the allocation of state funds under a variety of programmes. Census data may be used to monitor trends and conditions in a country or to compare them with those in other countries.

Census information is analysed and presented for the country as a whole and also for progressively smaller subdivisions, such as the provinces of South Africa or metropolitan areas in comparison to rural areas.

Any information furnished by individuals during the census is absolutely confidential and not available to any private or government agencies, except in the form of a summary of the statistical compilations.

5.9.1.2 *Vital statistics*

Vital statistics are the data collected for ongoing recording or registration of all births, adoptions, deaths, foetal deaths, marriages, divorces, legal separations and annulments. The community nurse should be familiar with these registration certificates and she should know where they can be obtained for the population with which she works.

(a) Registration of births

The registration of live births is one of the corner-stones in the system of vital statistics. It provides identification, which is essential for individuals as citizens. Proof of birth is required to obtain a passport, identity document or driver's licence, and for school entrance, immunisation or any other form of proof of identity.

(b) Registration of deaths

Death certificates provide information on the decedent's characteristics such as age, sex, race, occupation and also information on the conditions which led to death. This information is vitally important for epidemiologists as it may, for example, indicate at what age people die of a certain disease or what the mortality rate for a specific race, area or occupation is.

There are, however, many problems associated with information on the cause of death of a person:

- the amount of information available about the decedent will depend on the extent to which he had been treated medically before his death. For example, a person with a long history of carcinoma may have detailed medical records, but a healthy person who dies in an accident obviously will not have any medical history that could lead to or indicate the cause of his death;
- multiple causes are not indicated on a death certificate. The decedent may have several diseases contributing to his death, but under current procedure, only one cause is selected;
- the classification of the causes of death is not standardised; and
- procedural regulations inhibit and/or delay accurate and regular notifications of deaths, e.g. foetal or neonatal deaths.

5.9.1.3 *Morbidity data*

Through the systematic collection of morbidity data, disease rates can be determined in relation to time and place. Sources for data on morbidity include:

(a) Reports on notifiable diseases

Notifiable diseases are regulated under the Health Act. This list of diseases may be updated and changed according to the changes in health status of a specific country. Even the case definitions of disease may be changed. In 1994, for example, acute flaccid paralysis in children under the age of five was declared a notifiable condition in South Africa. In 1996, the risk population changed and the case definition was extended to include all children under the age of 15 years.

The notification of diseases is of great public health importance as it focuses the attention firstly on risk populations. This is of great importance in the surveillance and control of diseases. It is well known and documented that people living in overcrowded conditions are much more at risk of contracting tuberculosis, measles, or any other infectious disease. These people are then regarded as the risk population.

Secondly, notification of diseases serves as an evaluation model of control programmes. For example, the effectiveness of the national control programme for tuberculosis can be evaluated against the number of new cases reported.

A third purpose is to learn more about emerging problems or imminent epidemics, such as has been done by the surveillance of tuberculosis, where pro-active chemoprophylactic strategies were implemented.

There are specified legal guidelines for the notification of diseases in any country as well as for notification to the World Health Organisation.

Accurate notification of diseases depends on committed, informed and accurate health personnel, specifically doctors and nurses responsible for accurate differential diagnosis and the completion and processing of the necessary documentation.

(b) Other sources for statistics on morbidity patterns include:

- All kinds of hospital or/and clinic records such as road-to-health-charts, attendance registers of patients visiting the reproductive health clinics, theatre registers, casualty registers, discharge records and many more. Record keeping is often accused of "taking the nurse away from the patient". Effective record keeping should not be that time consuming. Patients and the community themselves could take co-responsibility for accurate record keeping and could be actively involved in collecting relevant data for specific studies. Regular evaluation of the value of specific records and statistics should be done and all record keeping and statistics that are not optimally used should be adapted or discarded.
- Records of private practitioners: all categories and all levels of specialisation.
- Records of insurance and medical aid schemes.

5.9.1.4 Responses to questionnaires

The use of questionnaires in obtaining data for epidemiological study is an important tool in determining the health or social status as well as perceptions, values, attitudes and health behaviour of the population.

5.9.1.5 *Household surveys*

Through the use of household surveys, information about the medical conditions and other pertinent social and personal characteristics are obtained. These surveys may indicate the health status in a community and may serve as a basis for determining priorities in the health-care policy of a population.

5.9.1.6 *Laboratory data*

Data obtained from laboratory studies are often reliable and valid and may serve as an important tool to epidemiologists in evaluating the extent and cause of a problem or to confirm and verify data collected in another way.

5.9.1.7 *Environmental monitoring*

Health hazards found in the environment are sometimes investigated by the government or other agencies. Usually the investigation concerns pollutants such as pesticides, industrial wastes, radioactive or nuclear materials, chemical pollutants, noise pollution and a variety of other health hazards.

5.9.2 Informal investigations

This is an area where every community nurse is directly involved. Informal inquiries are made about diseases and conditions in the clinic nearly every day to shed light on the reasons for a specific condition. The community nurse should, however, develop an analytic and detecting attitude as well as the ability to collate and coordinate a mass of information gained in an informal way into objective and measurable criteria.

5.9.3 Scientific studies

Formal epidemiological studies are often contracted to experts in the different fields of the health sciences. A multidisciplinary team approach is valuable.

5.10 SUMMARY

The science of epidemiology is not new. The use of epidemiology has led to the identification, prevention and control of many diseases. Nurses are important partners in all aspects of epidemiologic studies as well as in the implementation and evaluation of health-intervention strategies based on information gained through epidemiologic studies.

QUESTIONS

1. Discuss what is meant by the term "epidemiology".
2. Discuss the relationship between the epidemiological process and the nursing process.

3. Write short notes on the contribution of the community nurse to epidemiological research.
4. Describe tuberculosis as a community health problem in which you may use epidemiological investigation for primary prevention.
5. Calculate the infant mortality rate in Johannesburg in 1996 based on the records of 25 infant deaths and 1 468 live births during this same year.
6. Analyse the data and statistics that already exist in your workplace. Describe their value.

FURTHER READING

Clark, M.J. 1996. *Nursing in the community*. Norwalk, Connecticut: Appleton & Lange.

Last, J.M. 1987. *Public health and human ecology*. Norwalk, Connecticut: Appleton & Lange.

Spradley, B.W. 1996. *Community health nursing*. Boston: Little, Brown and Company.

Stanhope, M.E. & Lancaster, J. 1994. *Community health nursing: process and practice for promoting health*. St Louis: Mosby.

BIBLIOGRAPHY

Clark, M.J.D. 1984. *Community health care for today and tomorrow*. Reston: Prentice-Hall.

Last, J.M. 1987. *Public health and human ecology*. Norwalk, Connecticut: Appleton & Lange.

Spradley, B.W. 1996. *Community health nursing*. Boston: Little, Brown & Company.

Stanhope, M.E. & Lancaster, J. 1996. *Community health nursing: promoting health of aggregates, families and individuals*. 4th edition. St Louis: Mosby.

6 Community assessment

SUSAN HATTINGH

CHAPTER OBJECTIVES

After reading this chapter, the student should be able to:

- define the term "community assessment";
- explain the differences between geographically bound communities and socially bound communities;
- formulate guidelines on how to do a community assessment;
- explain the importance of a community assessment; and
- describe the community's participation in assessing a community.

6.1 INTRODUCTION

In South Africa with its highly complex social structure, which is not always easily understood, it is important that the community nurse should know and understand the needs and characteristics of the community in which she works. To achieve this understanding of the community, a community assessment must be carried out.

It is only through an objective assessment that one develops an awareness of the community's perceived needs and wants or desires in relation to the measured needs. The community assessment is undertaken to compile a health index of the community and ultimately to determine the health needs of that community. Through assessment of the community, health priorities are highlighted and services may be planned and rendered in accordance with these priorities so that the health status of the community can be improved.

Turner and Chavigny (1988:119) state that the idea behind the compilation of a community assessment is to determine the occurrence and distribution of selected environmental, socio-economic and behavioural conditions that affect disease control, as well as to promote health in a community.

A community assessment involves a team approach and collaboration between all role players. The community should be actively involved at all stages. The community nurse's role in the assessment is to empower the community to identify and where possible to solve its own health problems, to coordinate the planning and implementation of health intervention, to give continued support and guidance when necessary and to facilitate collaboration between individuals and groups to improve the total health of individuals and communities. The community nurse therefore needs to adapt and implement a non-directive approach. She should learn to respect different cultural views and practices on health and allow individuals and communities to take informed decisions and actions regarding their own health.

6.2 WHAT IS A COMMUNITY?

There are many and varied definitions of the term "community".

A community can be defined as a group of people in a defined geographical area with common goals and objectives and the potential for interacting with one another.

This group of people may be delimited by social or geographical boundaries. Some social communities may have the world as their geographical boundary, but all communities should be contextualised within boundaries. Some communities may have different and sometimes even clashing cultures and views, but communities cannot survive if they do not have common objectives such as respecting each other's privacy, allowing for differences between their members, etc. Individual behaviour within communities may have an effect on other individuals in the same community and/or on the environment within which the community lives.

According to the abovementioned definition, communities can therefore be small or large, e.g. all mothers with children under the age of five in South Africa or the children attending a small farm school or even the patients in a specific ward in a hospital.

The above definition is a more comprehensive one, but some definitions emphasise either the geographical boundaries of communities or the social boundaries and the resulting characteristics and functions of communities.

6.2.1 Geographically-bound communities

Geographically-bound communities are viewed by Burgess and Ragland (1983:124–125) as those communities with formal boundaries assigned by law, or with boundaries that have been recognised by local customs over time. These communities include places such as townships (e.g. Soweto, Mamelodi), cities (e.g. Cape Town, Durban), neighbourhoods (e.g. Sandton, Motherwell) or homelands (e.g. Bophuthatswana, Venda). The geographical boundaries can only be changed by legal procedures and usually with the consent of the community.

The health of a community is affected by its geographical location, the location of health services, the geographical features of the environment, the plants, animals and the man-made environment within its geographical boundaries.

Geographical boundaries have various functions:

- homogeneity is maintained, but heterogeneity is recognised;
- protection of residents is assured;

- a feeling of belonging exists among residents;
- funding and other assistance is allocated specifically to that community;
- the division of labour develops specifically in accordance with the needs of that community;
- specialised roles and co-operation are directed towards the uniqueness of that community; and
- social control is exercised over residents or members.

6.2.2 Socially-bound communities

The social boundaries of a community are the strong, all-encompassing normative systems that define how people live in a given area, how they are related to one another and how they fit into their social organisation. The members of a community know and interact with one another and their behaviour and attitudes are regulated by a set of norms, values and social institutions that have been adopted by the community as a whole. The social boundaries of a community are closely related to the culture and cultural system within a community.

Social boundaries may not necessarily be geographically defined. Groups within a community may attempt to perform communal functions to build social solidarity and to maintain a sense of belonging. The members of this community may be geographically scattered, but they have a certain feeling of belonging, which sustains the benefits of their association with that specific community. These communities are usually organised groups that share the same interests, views, needs, problems, norms or any other common feature. Socially-bound communities may be those communities with specific interests such as stamp collectors, or groups with special language and cultural interests, such as the Jewish community in Johannesburg.

The functions of social communities are as follows:

- there is a feeling of membership of a group or social system;
- identification with a specific group is assured;
- individuality is recognised;
- homogeneity is retained;
- members influence one another;
- social control is exercised over members to ensure conformity with norms;
- members are conscious of their roles and of the values of the group;
- a deep psychological and emotional relationship is formed;
- mostly close, intimate and personal ties bind people in the community;
- the expected behaviour of the individual is related to the social status or setting of the community;
- socialisation is exercised in this community;
- sanctions or penalties are imposed on those who deviate from the norms;
- traditional, ethnic and/or cultural characteristics are retained;
- there is a generalisation and maintenance of social solidarity and normative integration within the community;

- goods and services are delivered to serve the unique needs of the community;
- opportunities are provided and outlets for social participation are assured;
- mutual support of members is evident; and
- taxes or other funds are paid in aid of members.

A person may belong to more than one community at the same time. One may, for instance, live in Durban but belong to a cultural or other organisation in East London. Many socially bound communities have branches or sub-groups in various towns, cities or communities. The Nursing Association may be viewed as a socially bound community; only nurses may belong to this association. There is, however, the Community Health Association of South Africa to which anyone with an interest in the health sciences can belong, for example nurses, doctors, physiotherapists, herbalists, traditional healers, pharmacists, psychologists and any other individual or group that associates with the aims and objectives of that specific association. This particular association has an open membership. Thus if one belongs to any social group, it is regarded as a social community in which the activities of that group take place.

6.3 DEFINITION OF A COMMUNITY ASSESSMENT

A community assessment is regarded as the process by which the community's health status is evaluated through the collection of data on that community.

The assessment is usually done through descriptive epidemiology. Information is collected on a target community or a community at risk to describe its characteristics as well as the problems that are experienced in that community. The information that is obtained through the community assessment is used for the numerators of proportions and rates. The target community or the community at risk will form the denominator.

Community surveys are often conducted to determine the target or risk population and are then followed up by more in-depth and specific assessments of the risk groups.

6.4 TYPES OF COMMUNITY ASSESSMENT

Spradley (1991:155–61) suggests various types of community assessment: comprehensive assessment, familiarisation, problem-orientated assessment and community sub-system assessment.

6.4.1 Comprehensive assessment

This type of assessment seeks to discover all the relevant community information (as will be discussed later in this chapter). It is a complete study of the community and detailed data are collected. This type of community assessment is, however, expensive and time-consuming, and is always conducted within a team.

Because of the magnitude and costs involved, the value of such comprehensive assessments should be carefully considered.

6.4.2 Familiarisation

This is the most frequently used community assessment. It involves the study of readily available data on the community and the collection of specific and relevant first-hand data. A working knowledge of the community can thus be formed. For a newly appointed community nurse in a relatively unknown community, a familiarisation assessment could be very valuable. A nurse should, however, not unnecessarily repeat community assessments.

6.4.3 Problem-orientated assessment

This is the type of assessment that responds to a certain need or evaluates the effect of health intervention on a specific problem. The problem-orientated assessment begins with a single problem, after which the community is assessed in terms of that particular problem. It is commonly used when familiarisation is not sufficient and comprehensive assessment is too expensive.

6.4.4 Community sub-system assessment

This type of assessment is similar to a problem-orientated assessment, but the field of study will cover aspects other than health problems. The focus is placed on one single dimension of a sub-system within a community, e.g. the influence of the traditional healer in one specific culture or the perception of school children regarding nursing and nurses.

6.5 DATA COLLECTED FOR COMMUNITY ASSESSMENT

Data collection is the basis for community assessments, but is often the most difficult step. Health information in South Africa has often been inappropriate, unavailable and inaccurate. All members of the health team should realise the importance of accurate record keeping, and should be empowered with the necessary knowledge and skills for optimal utilisation and critical evaluation of health information.

All available methods (observation, interviews, analysis of documents, etc) and all possible sources should be exploited for relevant health information, e.g. insurance companies, magistrates' offices, ministers of religion, etc.

There are basically two types of data collected when compiling a community assessment:

- Specific data about the community or target group to be investigated may lead to information on the specific problems of a particular community, such as statistics on morbidity, mortality and fertility, health status, services in the community, the community's attitudes, views, priorities, the resources in the community, the identification of risk factors in the community, and the availability, type and education of the manpower in the community.

- General information about the community, which leads to the identification of the strengths and weaknesses in a specific community. This information may lead to the identification of problems and the factors that contribute to problems. These include the geography, topography and demographic characteristics, the social and economic conditions, the political structure of the community, the infrastructure, cultural practices and attitudes, the environmental conditions and the relationship of the community with the outside world.

6.6 THE OBJECTIVES OF A COMMUNITY ASSESSMENT

A community assessment forms the basis for planning, intervention and evaluation in a community.

Through the data collected in a community assessment, the community diagnosis can be made and planning, implementation and evaluation of programmes can follow to promote health and to resolve existing health problems in a specific community. The ultimate goal is to improve the quality of life of all individuals, groups and communities.

The community assessment provides an understanding of the nature, complexity and magnitude of a particular problem. By assessing the services in a community, the available health-related resources can be identified and their efficiency evaluated. This can also indicate the state of well-being in the community.

Policy-makers can be made aware of the problems in a community and priorities can be established to resolve problems that have been identified.

It should, however, again be emphasised that a community assessment is not valid or possible without the participation of the community members. Planning or change of any aspect in a community is not possible without the knowledge, participation and the active involvement of the community. It is essential to determine the specific needs of a community as any aspects of planning revolve around the community's unique needs.

Without the knowledge of the dynamics in a community, recognition and acknowledgement of a health need by the community and a commitment to meet these needs, no change can take place. It is also important to distinguish between measured needs as opposed to perceived needs and wants in communities.

By assessing the community, cultural differences and traditions can be identified in relation to consumer concerns, needs, interests, strengths and motivations. Through this assessment the community nurse may develop an

FIGURE 6.1: An holistic approach to community assessment

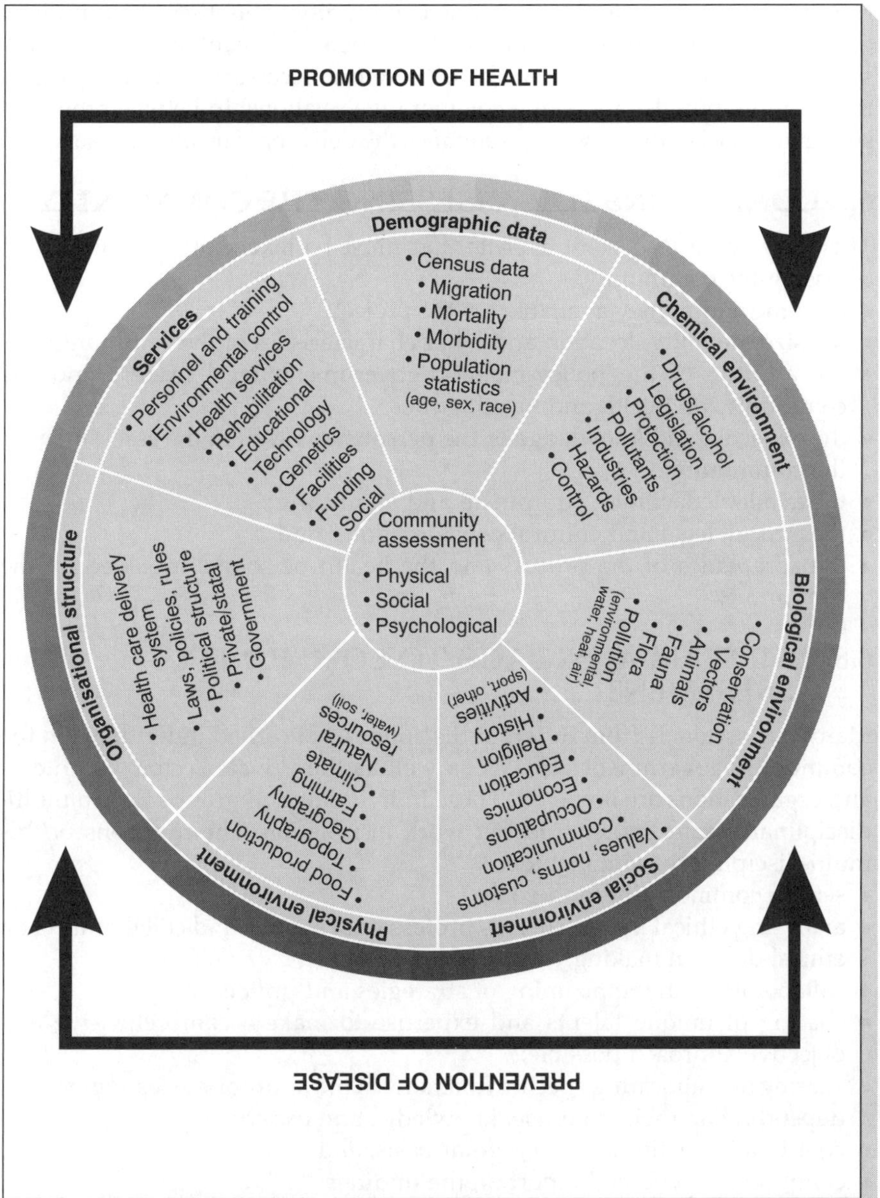

awareness of the community's perceptions of health, and of their values, attitudes and beliefs towards health. This information allows the nurse and other health professionals to plan acceptable and effective health activities and programmes.

One cannot generalise about communities, because health needs and resources are not consistent from one community to another. Assumptions cannot be made about any community's response to health care delivery. A systematic community assessment is therefore necessary, not only to gain information, but also to form a collaborative relationship between the consumer and the health provider to enhance the delivery of health-care services.

6.7 CONDITIONS FOR ASSESSING THE COMMUNITY

There are some important aspects that must be taken into account when assessing the community:

- the time and money available for the project;
- the size, mobility, location and other characteristics of the community;
- the attitude of the policy-makers, government, local leaders and the community on health and health issues;
- the expertise and knowledge of the persons involved in the assessment of the community;
- the available facilities, equipment and manpower;
- the ethical, legal and cultural considerations; and
- the acceptance of the process and the health personnel involved by the community.

6.8 THE TEAM APPROACH TO COMMUNITY ASSESSMENT

Many professionals from different disciplines, concerned individuals in the community, government officials as well as the private sector, volunteers and organisations are involved. These individuals and groups form a multi-disciplinary team that should not work in isolation. The functions of this multi-disciplinary team include:

- setting common aims and goals;
- analysing ethical issues, such as professional secrecy and collaborating on ethical decision making;
- collaborating on the planning of strategies and protocols;
- sharing of unique talents and expertise to make a comprehensive and objective approach possible;
- sharing and allocating specific functions to the appropriate team members depending on their expertise, knowledge and experience;
- coordinating activities on a regular basis; and
- compiling a combined report on the findings.

6.9 THE PROCESS OF COMMUNITY ASSESSMENT

The community assessment process consists of various steps, i.e. setting of aims or goals, data collection, collation and analysis of data, community diagnosis, planning, intervention and evaluation. Together these steps form

FIGURE 6.2: Sharing in a multi-disciplinary team

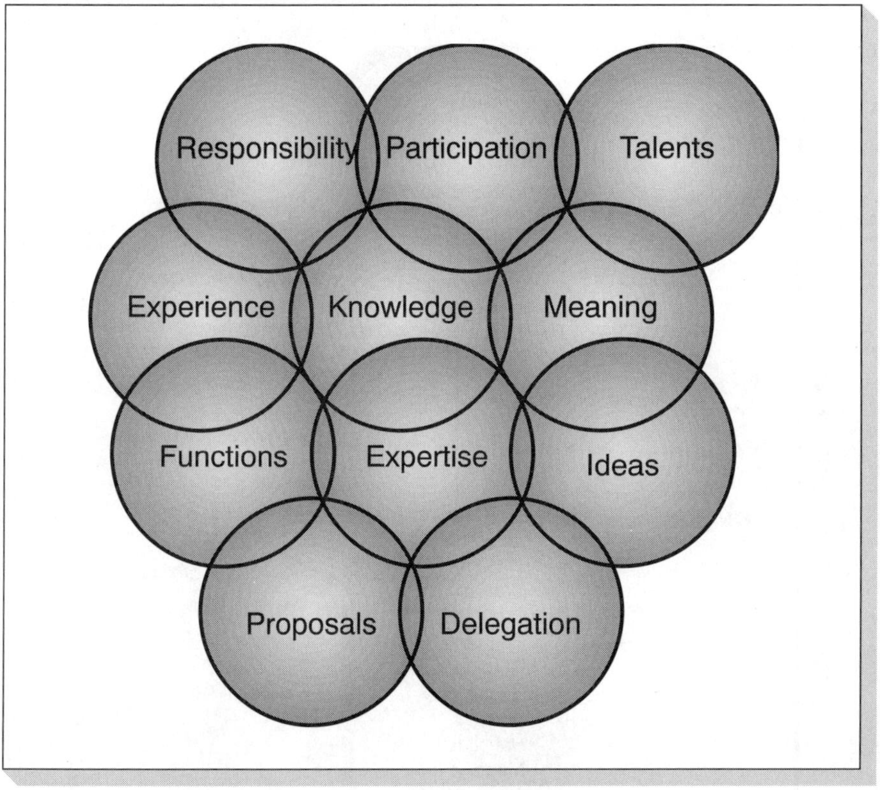

a logical, systematic and practical analysis of the community as a whole regarding a matter of concern to the community nurse. Empowering the community actively to participate, to take informed decisions and to initiate strategies to meet its own health needs are aspects that should be integrated throughout the process. How this involvement and empowerment should be done will depend on aspects such as:

- the urgency, extent and type of the need;
- the number and group of the community affected;
- the attitudes and values of the community;
- the acceptance of health intervention strategies by the communities; and
- the available resources.

Community nurses are usually an integral part of the community, are well informed, sensitive to the needs of the community and are well accepted by the community. They therefore have a specific coordinating and facilitating role to play in this regard.

FIGURE 6.3: A comprehensive community assessment approach

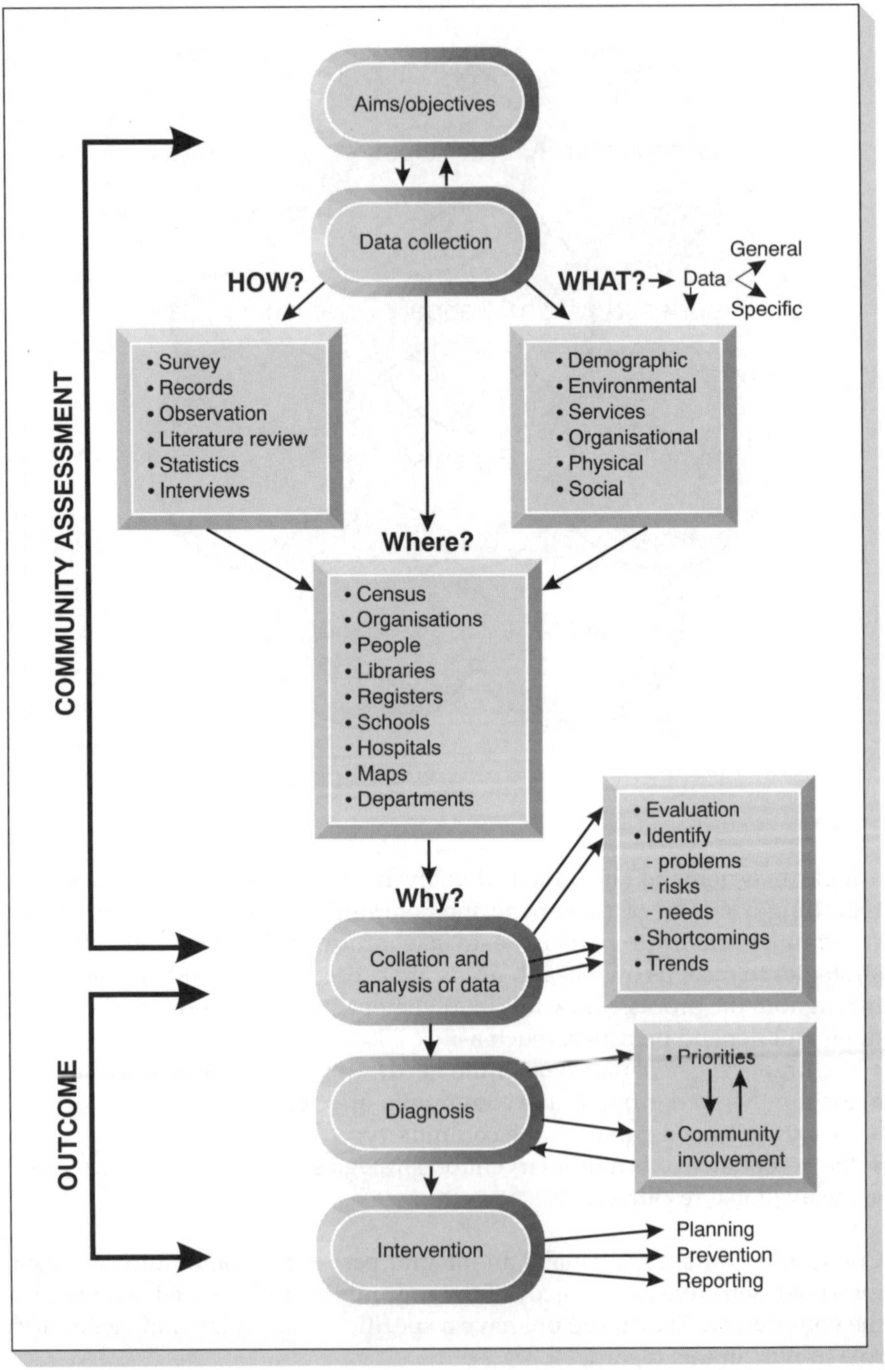

6.9.1 Setting of aims or goals

The setting of aims or goals is the starting point in the process of community assessment. These aims and goals will vary according to the population to be studied. Aims and goals are the precise statements of the desired outcome and are carefully determined to suit the priorities of a community.

The setting of objectives involves collaboration between the health team, the community and the officials involved with the community, and this process may involve considerable negotiation. It is therefore recommended that the community nurse who deals with this kind of negotiation should have a knowledge of community problems, legislation and other relevant matters concerning the problem to be assessed. An experienced nurse with a keen interest and a responsible outlook should be the person to be assigned this task.

6.9.2 Data collection

A knowledge of the various components that exist in a community (for example, the economic, political, health, population, organisational elements, etc.), is essential for community health.

The assessment team uses the data to diagnose, plan, implement and evaluate the health situation in the community. There are basically three questions that could be asked when collecting data:

- What will be collected?
- How will it be collected?
- By whom will it be collected?

6.9.2.1 *What will be collected?*

(a) Demographic attributes and population characteristics

There are a number of demographic features of the community to be assessed. The size, sex, race and population density of the community are its most important biological features. This may reflect the genetic features, environmental origin, socio-cultural features, interests of groups, needs of different groups and various other specific factors relevant to diseases and/or conditions in the community.

- The racial and ethnic composition of a community has important implications. There are certain diseases and conditions that are common to certain race groups. It is therefore important not only to look at the ethnic-racial make-up, but also to identify the implications of this make-up for the health and stability of a community.
- Statistics on morbidity, mortality and fertility reflect the growth or decline patterns in the community. Population changes place extreme demands on the provision of health services. Any fluctuation in the population size affects the health of the entire community. A decline in the community, such as the depopulation of rural areas (for example, as seen in some towns

in the Eastern Cape) poses a serious threat to the health of those who stay behind, as economic and living conditions may decline.

- Stability in a community is reflected by the mobility and changes within it and census data give a clear indication of how frequently people move, what the rates of immigration and emigration are and whether refugees contribute to a changing factor in the community. The influx of immigrants to a population may cause cultural conflict or competing demands for resources, jobs and services. Major changes in the demographic structure over relatively short periods of time give a clear indication of the possible problems experienced by a community. This may be seen, for example, when members of the community are drafted into the army or when migrant workers have to go to their place of employment.
- Rates can be compared to national statistics and to communities of comparable size, as well as other countries. This comparison will give health professionals an idea of the general health of the community, the types of services needed and the significant health problems.
- Migrant seasonal workers, students and tourists place a demand on the immediate resources of a community. The effects of their presence should be carefully recorded to detect how they influence the local stable community and its resources.
- The educational level of a community is of great importance as this reflects the level of dependence of individuals, and the socio-economic contribution and technological progress of the community.
- Employment and unemployment figures give an indication of the number of people who are professional, non-professional or unemployed. The dependence on national financial resources can thus be determined and this may reflect the health and socio-economic status of the community. A high unemployment rate will influence tax payments and this forms a vicious circle of social, psychological, physical and environmental problems that affect the entire community.

(b) The attributes of the physical environment

The environment in which a community lives consists of physical, social and psychological elements. These elements interact with one another and are inseparable. A change or event in one necessarily affects the others.

The health of a community directly affects all the members of a community directly. For example, a high population growth in a poor community with limited physical resources such as water, sanitation, food, housing, etc. will have a direct effect on the health and well-being of the entire community. In an environment of heavily polluted air, it can be expected that the health of that specific community will be adversely affected. An example could be a mining community where asbestos may be a threat to the health of the entire community.

Data about the physical environment include the following:

- Whether this community can be regarded as a rural, urban or suburban community, because each of these communities may experience its own unique problems. For example, the rural community may experience problems with regard to the availability of health services.
- The size of the community has a direct impact on the availability of resources. Whether the community has a high or low density, there are specific problems and needs associated with health provision and service in each case. Understanding the composition of a community is an important early step in determining the level of health in a community.
- Climate, climatic changes and weather conditions may all affect the health and safety of the people residing in the community. For example, in the tropics heat-related diseases are encountered, and in winter, poor weather conditions and snow in the mountainous areas of Lesotho affect the local population who are cut off from all sources of food, fuel, health services and other resources.
- Housing conditions often reveal a great deal about the community. For example, overcrowding and slum areas may give an indication of the type of people living in that particular community. Their interests, resources, stability and their attitudes towards the maintenance of their environment are frequently indicated by their housing conditions.
- Sanitation and disposal of wastes and the hazards experienced or associated with these, as well as other environmental controls operating in the area, including air, water pollution and so on, all affect the health of the community.
- The water supply is a prime indicator of health in the community. For example, the nurse should consider whether the community obtains its water from wells, rivers or unprotected dams, what the fluoride content is, what the levels of contamination are, and what the availability of this important resource is.
- Potential disasters which may be expected by a community could have a bearing on its health. These include either man-made or natural disasters such as potential floodings, cyclones or living near nuclear plants.
- Vectors, such as insects found in the area, may be the cause of many diseases. Flies, mosquitoes and vermin are vectors that could spread disease.
- Pollution, such as noise, heat and smoke, affects levels of health.
- Mining activities should be noted, as major food supplies could be contaminated by these activities. Some mining activities also pose a threat to the health and lives of their employees and the people in the surrounding community.
- The potential for accidents in a community should be noted. For example, the conditions of the roads should be assessed, and the community should be made aware of unprotected swimming-pools or rivers in which children could drown.

- Good channels of communication, such as the radio and telephone, are essential for providing effective health care in a community.
- Animals on nearby farms such as dairy or pig farms may provide insect breeding grounds and be offensive to the community. Animals may carry dangerous infectious diseases. It is not uncommon for dogs infected with rabies to attack people in the community. This aspect should be assessed by the community nurse.
- Fauna and flora found in the community may indicate what the people eat and what their outlook on conservation is. They also give an indication of the climate of the area. Poisonous plants and disease-carrying animals may affect the health of a community. Plants that are not indigenous to this country may pose a threat to a community because they might occupy valuable land that could be used for food production, pose a fire hazard or reduce grazing land for both domestic and wild animals. Plants such as the Kariba weed, a free-floating fern found in freshwater, form a thick carpet on the water's surface, increasing the chance of severe flooding and reducing the amount of drinking water available to the community. It also provides a breeding ground for mosquitoes and bilharzia-carrying snails. In addition, it kills fish that could have been used as a good source of food.
- Nature conservation is closely related to the abovementioned aspects and some people measure the level of civilisation of communities by the extent to which they conserve their environment for future generations.
- Agriculture is an important part of the environment and lies at the heart of a country's well-being. In times of severe drought, floods or any other natural disaster, war and violence, the health and socio-economic status of the community is affected because of a lack of income from agricultural products, production and protection of food sources. This is associated with a loss of income, jobs and self-esteem for those who work in the agricultural and associated sectors. Some uncontrolled or incorrect agricultural practices may influence the community's potential to produce food. The environment may be altered by these agricultural practices, resulting in soil erosion which, in turn, may have disastrous effects on a community.
- Protection services, such as the location and activities of the police or other services rendered to protect the community, their belongings and the environment, should also be taken into account. A stable community is a safe and healthy community. Homicide rates may provide an indication of stability in relation to safety in the community.
- Transport facilities in the community are important because they indicate the mobility of the community and its ability to get to and from health services. It is particularly important to assess the availability of transport for children and older or physically handicapped persons.
- The community's access to stores and shopping areas, their size, location and trading hours should be noted. The type of stores found in a

community may reflect its interests and resources – they could also reflect a community's tourist potential. The presence of tourists in a community also contributes to its financial well-being, as they bring money into that community.

- The geographical boundaries of the community serve as an indication for measuring the patterns of disease and the spread of disease. Communities are related to other communities and can therefore be compared with one another.

The physical features of a community affect many aspects of life. They determine the prevalence of certain diseases, conditions or specific problems. The physical environment may affect many things within the community, for example transport, the kind of food grown, types of industry, the presence of mines and the type of illness or health needs that affect the members of that community.

(c) The attributes of the psychological environment

Data about the psychological environment include the following:

- Exposure to stress may increase the danger of cardiovascular diseases, suicide and other stress-related problems.
- Violence and gang activities in the community should be assessed as these factors may bring about many problems in a community and cause stress, injury and death.
- The availability and use or misuse of alcohol, drugs or other substances have a psychological effect on the community.
- The norms and values of the community contribute to its psychological climate. Activities such as prostitution may reflect the norms of the community.
- The relationship between family members and the occurrence of divorce, child abuse and abuse of the elderly all point to the psychological health of the community.
- Behavioural patterns in the community, such as homosexuality, illegitimacy and criminal abortions also cause stress.
- The attitudes of the community will be reflected in its general health status – a negative or apathetic attitude towards addressing community problems may have a severe effect on the general health status of the community and on the prosperity of the country as a whole.

(d) The attributes of the social environment

Every community has a social system of dynamic, unique quality and each community should be viewed in relation to its social environment. The social environment includes the following:

- The responsibility of the governing body and power structure of the community and their participation in health matters in the community.

- The formal leadership structure in the community.
- Income is related to socio-economic status, employment, educational levels and attitudes towards self-care in the community.
- Social class gives an indication of both the socio-economic states and educational level of the individuals or groups in the community. Spradley (1991) relates that the members of the upper class in a community are usually rich, well-educated, have good jobs and are powerful. Lower-class people tend to be poor, uneducated, have a low self-esteem, live on insubstantial incomes and are less powerful. People with higher education tend to be physically healthier and have a more positive attitude to life.
- Educational levels, the availability of schools as well as attendance and attitudes towards education are an important part of the social environment. Informal and traditional education play an important role in socialising the individual in his own community and within his own culture. The educational system is part of the overall social system in a community and goes hand in hand with the socio-economic level and health of the individual, and the total well-being of the community. The literacy level of a community determines its level of civilisation. Educational facilities include all those facilities from pre-schools, primary schools, high schools, colleges, technikons, technical colleges and universities. The number and type of educational facilities available in the community reflect the priorities and interests of the community members.
- Marital status will indicate the stability of the community.
- Family composition and other family characteristics specific to the community need to be taken into account, for example extended family patterns and cultures that allow more than one wife.
- Religion and religious affiliations and beliefs influence health, for example ideas on family planning and food taboos.
- Recreation and sporting facilities and programmes that enhance recreational participation should all be assessed – there may be no competition, poor facilities and little motivation or interest. There are also risks associated with recreation and leisure pursuits, for example injuries may be sustained during rugby, motor sport and water sport, and shooting accidents among those who hunt for recreation. Recreation is important for the physical and mental health of a community, and also plays a role in the socialisation of its members. One must determine whether there are facilities for all age groups, and one should also assess the quality, type of recreation, the hours in which recreation is available and the attendance and interest shown in these recreational facilities.
- Languages spoken in the community will affect the health education as well as the expressions and perceptions of health and health-related matters. Language barriers cause cultural sensitivities that would need to be taken into consideration when planning health education and intervention.

- Cultural diversity may influence health practices and attitudes and will influence the behaviour of the individuals in a community. For example, a community's views on diseases, traditional remedies and practices, its belief in the traditional healer, and the value it places on health, life and death are all determined by culture. In a country with a diverse ethnicity, such as Southern Africa, these cultural values must be assessed, studied and, above all, respected by the health profession.
- The availability of shopping and other facilities contributes to a community's social environment.
- Communication networks and media (including newspapers, publications, radio, television, meetings and telephones) make an important contribution to the social environment. The type of written media available in a community will depend on the educational level of its members. Newspapers give priority to politics and major events that take place in a community and thus provide insight into community life. They also provide valuable information on what goes on in other parts of the world. However, the media must never be regarded as absolute because they are subject to bias, misinterpretations and error.
- Political systems and structure in the community will determine the stability, provision of services, freedom of individuals and groups, and the general well-being and safety of the community. In a country where there are opposing and warring parties one can expect political instability, which will in turn affect the health of the community.
- Informal power structures in the community should be identified. They may include youth gangs or even a clustering of customers of a neighbourhood bar. Keen observational skills are required to identify the informal power structures and how they affect community life.
- Voluntary organisations should be identified and their activities in the community noted. These organisations include, among others, the Red Cross, Rotary and Lions Club International. Their participation and involvement in the community should not be underestimated.
- Safety in the community, particularly in relation to the services provided by the police, ambulance and fire department, is extremely important. The location of these protection services and the trust that the community puts in them should be evaluated. Safety in the community can also be measured against the frequency of victimisation, criminal offences, traffic violations, murders, assaults, child abuse and rape. One must detect whether community members feel safe and whether they are conscious of their safety and the safety of their fellow members in the community. In some communities crime prevention programmes are initiated and units are formed through the participation of the community.
- Social problems such as alcoholism, suicide and abuse should be addressed, as they may be the cause of social disintegration in a community.

- The historic heritage of a community gives it its character and determines how groups, individuals and the whole community identify with the historic past. There are certain symbols, rituals and historic contingencies that are unique to a specific community. These historic events or contingencies affect the outlook, values and interests of that community.
- The availability and accessibility of services in the community, their strengths and limitations should also be studied.

(e) Socio-economic features

The socio-economic features of a community have implications for both the level of health and the ability of the community to pay for the necessities of life. One cannot sustain life without the means to do so. These means come in the form of economic assets. The health of each individual and family will affect the entire community. For example, a large population of elderly persons with a limited income must be provided for by the community in which they live. This can drain the economic resources of that community.

It is important for the assessment team to know the range of income levels of the members of the community it serves, as this will help to understand the community's needs for different services and whether these services should be private or government subsidised. The socio-economic features of a community also indicate the type of facilities, housing and interests of a community. Certain diseases can also be attributed to socio-economic standards, for example obesity or malnutrition.

Persons of different income levels live in different areas and this can indicate their living standard, values, interests, outlooks and goals in life. Overcrowding has been found to lead to the increase of certain diseases such as measles, tuberculosis and scabies, and also to stress-related conditions such as suicide, abuse of alcohol and drugs, violence and rape.

All developments that may affect the socio-economic status of a community are assessed, for example industrial development may play an important role in the overall socio-economic structure of a community.

(f) Health systems

Information on the types, availability, accessibility, effectiveness and use or underuse of health services is of vital importance in the assessment of the community. The assessment team should assess the preventative services available in the community on a primary, secondary and tertiary level.

Stumbling blocks in the way of the delivery of these services should be pointed out

The referral system within the community should be assessed. For example, the nurse should be aware of the referral possibilities for people with psychological problems, suspected AIDS cases or any other specialised problem.

FIGURE 6.4: Information collected in a community

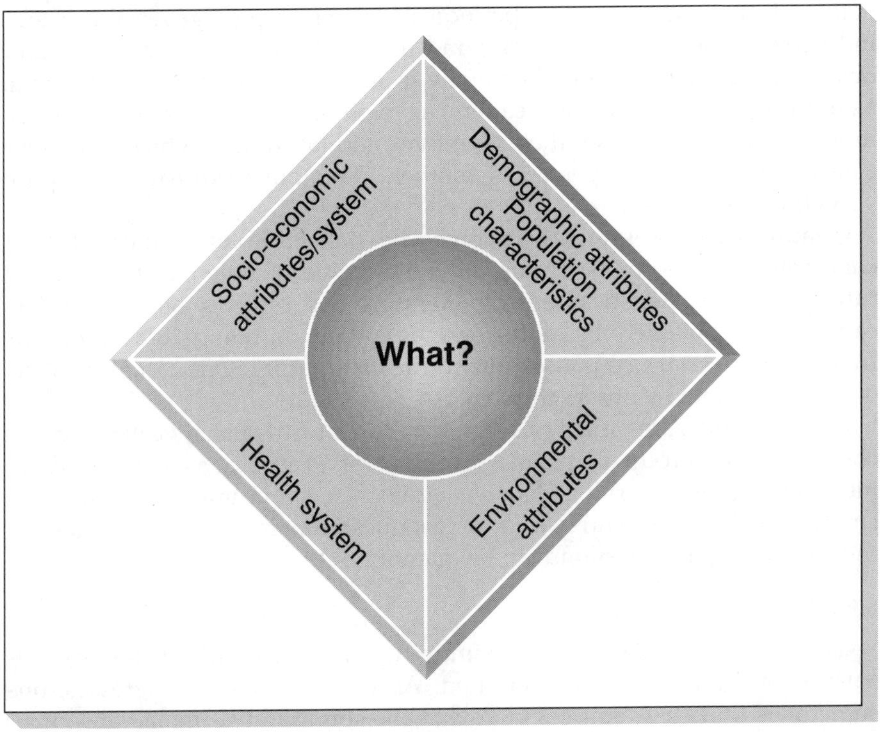

The assessment team must have a clear understanding of all the systems in a community. It must be known what they are, how they interact and what their goals are. It is important to note the level of sophistication of the health-care delivery system within a particular community.

If health information on a specific aspect is not available, the assessment team should determine the importance of the information and what to do about the problem.

6.9.2.2 How will the data be collected?

The selection of methods for collecting data in the process of community assessment is vital if the aims of the assessment are to be accomplished. A variety of methods can be used as indicated in Figure 6.4. Different methods of data collection give different types of information.

The particular method of data collection selected will depend on the type of community chosen to study, the funds available, the time to complete the project and the people involved in the assessment. Qualitative approaches focus on the examination of perceptions of health, attitudes and health concerns, as voiced by the members of a community. Qualitative data are data expressed in words rather than in numbers. Information can be gathered from newspapers, periodicals, films, tapes, government and industrial records, private diaries and books of many kinds. Surveys and observations are used most frequently in the collection of qualitative data. Community members and leaders as well as key informants can be interviewed to establish their opinions and attitudes, which can vary considerably from one person to another. Qualitative assessments require vast clinical expertise.

Quantitative assessments involve the collection of numerical data concerning events in the community. This type of data can be obtained through census, statistics, records, literature and reviews. Numerical data can also be obtained by doing surveys and compiling figures on the frequency of certain responses within the community. One can also collect quantitative data by observation.

A community assessment can simply take the form of an investigation of a community or group of people through, for example, asking questions, interviewing or observing. However, when a community assessment is conducted along these lines, a consistent questionnaire must be used so that the answers to the questions can be quantified for computer analysis.

6.9.2.3 Sources of data

Before an assessment of the community can be conducted, the various sources of data should be identified. As the assessment progresses, one sometimes finds new sources of data in the community. The list of sources where data can be obtained for community assessment given in this chapter is not exhaustive - the unique characteristics of a community should always be kept in mind and therefore sources of data will often depend on the particular features of the community.

- Census data supply information on the demographic and population characteristics of a community.
- Various health departments supply information on health-care facilities or disease patterns.
- Libraries can contribute to information on the history of a community and yearbooks usually supply important information on the characteristics of a community.
- Registers of births and deaths, certain diseases such cancer, or conditions such as organic phosphate poisoning, can be of great value.
- Various state departments will provide specialised data, for example the Department of Agriculture can supply information on agricultural conditions, soil erosion and pollution.
- Schools may supply information such as the level of immunisation, teenage pregnancies and the use of drugs in schools.
- Police and other prominent public services are valuable sources of information on accidents, crime rates and violations of traffic rules.

- Area maps may indicate the size and boundaries of a community. For example, Lebowa, a homeland of the Sotho nation, is situated on the border with Mozambique, a war-torn country where famine is rife. This influences the internal structure of the Lebowa community as thousands of refugees must be accommodated.
- Directories such as the Yellow Pages and various other information services can be consulted to get information on services available in the community.
- Local and provincial services keep various forms of information on a large number of aspects in a community, such as housing, schools, clinics and demographics.
- Hospitals and clinics supply valuable information on diseases, operations and conditions treated, which can indicate the health status of a community.
- Key persons in the community should never be disregarded. These people may be in an official capacity or they may have no official status. For example, valuable historical information can be obtained from older family members or acquaintances who have lived in the specific community for a long time.
- Private organisations, for example the National Occupational Safety Association, can provide an indication of the safety and occupational hazards in industry.
- Industries keep health records that may be examined.
- Organisations such as Operation Hunger and others supply information about immediate and long-term needs and problems. Other important associations, such as the Cancer Association and Cripple Care Association, have an important role to play in the provision of data on a community.
- Professional organisations, associations and other professional bodies, for example the Nursing Association, may supply information on the attitudes and activities of the community nurses, and the manpower provision in various services.

It must, however, always be remembered that some data can only be collected by means of observation of and interviews with the community or the target group.

Documentation forms an integral part of the whole community assessment and should therefore be decided upon by the assessment team, standardised and meticulously and accurately completed. A file should be kept so that it can be referred to when necessary, and it should be regularly updated.

6.9.2.4 Practical tips

Here are some practical tips that should be considered when assessing the community:

- make a tour of the community to get the "feel" of the place;

- note sites and make notes of where you want to return to;
- devise a plan of action;
- delegate tasks, but ensure that the person(s) to whom you delegate is informed and empowered;
- set time limits;
- take photographs, slides, movies and videos if possible;
- make appointments – never go unannounced as officials will not see you;
- when making appointments, state reasons so that the person you want to see can be prepared;
- always give a clear indication of what information you want;
- arrive prepared – if you are not, you waste your own time and that of the person interviewed;
- attend community meetings to learn about the community;
- document all findings immediately or record them on a tape recorder;
- be objective at all times – test your objectivity and the validity and reliability of your findings with other knowledgable persons or groups; and
- ensure that professional secrecy and other ethical aspects are maintained at all times.

6.9.3 The collation and analysis of data

Once the data have been gathered, conclusions can be drawn and the following aspects of the community can be identified:

- general strengths;
- shortcomings and deficiencies;
- major social or economic problems;
- major health-related problems;
- risks;
- needs;
- wants; and
- current and proposed community action for problem solving.

The investigator should differentiate between those problems that she discovers herself and those that the community identifies. It has been found that something which, from the investigator's perspective, seems to be a problem in a community, may not necessarily be a priority to the community. The primary purpose of the community nurse should be to identify the strengths, weaknesses and deficiencies in a community. Once the health-care delivery system has been examined, she can then detect the shortcomings and needs that interfere with the preventative health approach.

Only when the community as a whole has been analysed can the true needs of the consumer be reflected and preventative measures be applied. Prevention is often overlooked when community problems are analysed and health services developed. This is because many health professionals have a curative rather than a preventative outlook on health.

Through collation and the analysis of data obtained in the community, the existing structures, attitudes and problems can be evaluated. Problems in the community can be identified and any vulnerability pointed out. Once the needs of the community have been identified, the shortcomings can be brought to the attention of the authorities. Data from other communities can be compared with a specific target community and the trends can be compared with one another. For example, the prevalence of measles in an urban and a rural community can be compared, as can death or fertility rates in different race groups and disease patterns in male and females in a community. One can also assess how income and educational levels compare, and what the relation between unemployment and suicide is.

The health services available to a community can be evaluated through the collation and analysis of the data. The problems, needs and shortcomings can be identified and the various services can be compared to one another, for example, the provision and training of manpower can be compared to other services. It is through pinpointing the strengths in the community that problems can be solved.

6.9.4 Community diagnosis

Once the assessment data have been obtained and organised, a clear statement of the problem should be formulated by formulating a community diagnosis.

6.9.5 Setting of priorities

Once the community diagnosis has been derived, priorities must be assigned for intervention. The health team, health care authorities, community leaders and the community as a whole must set priorities that will allow them the best use of available resources.

There are certain criteria identified by Clark (1996:417–20) that are used to set health-care priorities in a community. These include the following:

- the severity and the degree of the threat to the health of the community must be evaluated;
- the extent to which meeting one need depends on meeting other needs;
- the degree of concern about problems identified by the community;
- the extent to which the identified problems are able to be solved;
- the need for special educational measures related to the problems identified; and
- the extent to which additional resources and policies are needed.

It should always be remembered that the community is a vital link in the setting of priorities. Nothing can be achieved in a community without its active involvement and participation. The priorities set will be influenced by the value that the community places on health.

FIGURE 6.5: The community diagnosis

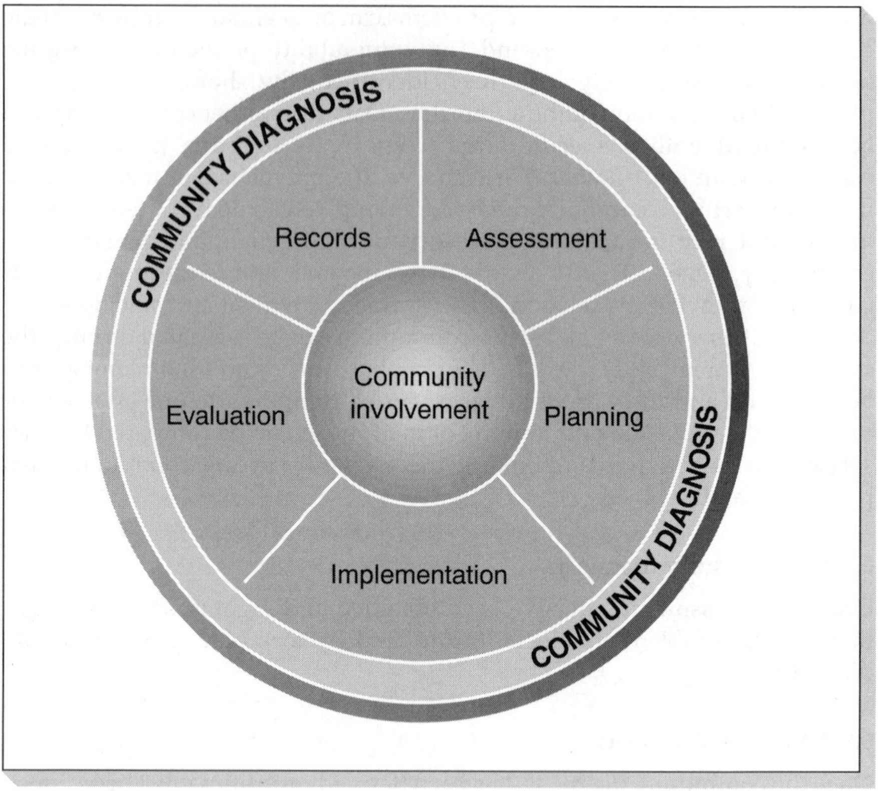

6.9.6 Planning

Once the community diagnosis has been established, planning objectives can be developed to prioritise and meet the needs of the community.

In the planning phase, the health team, together with the community, categorises the various risk factors that have been identified through demographic findings, characteristics of the community, socio-economic aspects, inherited and biological characteristics, and the physical conditions and environmental aspects that influence the community.

Problems are prioritised into short-range, mid-range and long-range goals and objectives. It is during this planning phase that the programme objectives are formulated. These objectives will clearly determine the extent to which the plan is expected to change the health problems of the community. The health professionals and the community must reach an agreement on the specific time-limit placed on the implementation of the professed plan and must agree on the extent to which changes will take place in the health system. There should also be absolute agreement between professionals, the governing bodies (both local and central) and the community on what should change.

It is essential that both professionals and local representatives of the community are involved so that they can arrive at a plan together to meet the community's particular health needs. As each plan must fit the community's own politics and power structure, the participation of local representatives is important. Professionals must not assume that the needs of one community are the same as the needs and priorities of another. All planning must, therefore, be realistic and congruent with the specific community's unique personality to be successful.

6.9.7 Intervention

Creativity is an essential part of the implementation phase. In this phase professional knowledge and judgement are shared to bring about change in the health status of the community. This change is inevitable and must be anticipated.

One must, however, keep in mind that intervention should take place within limits. Change may cause anxiety among the members of a community and as a result they may put up some resistance which could be hard to break down. It is a good policy to introduce the plan in different stages, so that severe or drastic change does not happen all at once but at a slower, more gradual pace.

It should be remembered that careful preparation for change, conscientious maintenance and effective communication should form the basis for negotiations between professionals and the community. Consistent respect of the views of others, rewards in the form of recognition of the community's views and an open approach without hidden agendas all help to minimise resistance to change, limit suspicion and contribute to the success of the plan.

6.9.8 Evaluation

In the evaluation phase, one must carefully examine the health care that has been provided both in terms of financial efficiency and the achievement of better health in the community. It is in the evaluation phase that one refers back to the goals and objectives formulated in the planning stage to determine if these goals and objectives have been met.

6.10 SUMMARY

This chapter has outlined the basic foundation of a community assessment. It has dealt with the data that need to be collected, the uses to which the data can be put, and it has demonstrated how to reach a nursing diagnosis.

The information provided here on community assessment is by no means exhaustive. The community nurse will find that each community is unique and has its own character. It is therefore impossible to make generalisations when conducting a community assessment.

QUESTIONS

1. Define the following concepts:
   (a) community
   (b) geographically-bound communities
   (c) socially-bound communities
   (d) community assessment
   (e) community diagnosis.
2. Discuss the purpose of a community assessment.
3. Describe the process of making a community assessment.
4. Formulate guidelines for implementing a community assessment and diagnostic activities in the practical setting.
5. Discuss ways in which a community nurse could facilitate community participation

FURTHER READING

Bullogh, B. & Bullogh V., 1990. *Nursing in the community.* St Louis: Mosby.

Burgess, W. & Ragland, E.C. 1983. *Community health nursing philosophy, process, practice.* Norwalk, Connecticut: Appleton-Century-Crofts.

Clark, M.J. 1996. *Nursing in the community.* Norwalk, Connecticut: Appleton & Lange.

Clemen-Stone, S., Eigsti, D.G. & McGuire, S.L. 1991. *Comprehensive family and community health nursing.* 3rd edition. St Louis: Mosby.

Spradley, B.W. 1996. *Community health nursing, concepts and practice.* Glenview, Illinois: Scott, Foresman and Company.

Turner, J.G. & Chavigny, K.H. 1988. *Community health nursing: an epidemiological perspective through the nursing process.* Philadelphia: Lippincott.

BIBLIOGRAPHY

Burgess, W. & Ragland, E.C. 1983. *Community health nursing philosophy, process, practice.* Norwalk, Connecticut: Appleton-Century-Crofts.

Clark, M.J. 1996. *Nursing in the community.* 2nd edition. Norwalk, Connecticut: Appleton & Lange.

Spradley, B.W. 1996. *Readings in community health nursing.* 4th edition. Philadelphia: Lippincott.

Turner, J.G. & Chavigny, K.H. 1988. *Community health nursing: an epidemiological perspective through the nursing process.* Philadelphia: Lippincott.

7 Aspects of health planning at primary health care level

MARGUERITE LOCK

LEARNING OBJECTIVES

Having studied this chapter, the health care provider at primary health care level should be able to:

- define health care planning and identify the basic requirements for effective planning at primary health care level;
- identify the impact that changing health approaches have had on health care planning;
- briefly discuss selected planning models;
- briefly discuss the steps in the health planning process; and
- discuss the role of the community nurse as a member of a health planning team.

7.1 INTRODUCTION

Health planning is an activity that facilitates informed decision-making when changes have to be made to meet identified health and health care needs within society both now and in the future. The planning process as a health-planning activity also provides a logical format for the analysis of a wide range of factors that could have either a negative or a positive impact on these planned changes.

7.2 HEALTH PLANNING AND CHANGING HEALTH ENVIRONMENTS

All over the world, health environments have changed substantially during the last quarter of this century. To appreciate the complexity of health planning today, it is therefore appropriate briefly to trace some of the major changes that have taken place in health environments and that have affected the planning process.

7.2.1 Health care environments from 1900 to 1955

Until the latter part of the 1950s, the health environment remained relatively uncomplicated. In the organisation of health services, a medical model dominated in which emphasis was given to the treatment and cure of diseases. Medical and nursing care was provided on an individual basis in hospitals, clinics, the consulting rooms of general practitioners and in homes. During this period, relatively few facilities were available for promotive, preventive and rehabilitative health care, and during this time the number of hospitals and clinics remained small.

The health team, made up primarily of the doctor, nurse and pharmacist, was clearly identified, as were the tasks and roles they were expected to fulfil. The career opportunities available were straightforward and followed a logical sequence, with few differentiated positions being identified. Changes took place at a slow pace and, in most instances, could be predicted. Health planning in this climate tended to be re-active, rather than pro-active, was seldom coordinated and generally took place in government environments.

7.2.2 Health care environments from 1955 to 1975

During the period of the late 1950s, 1960s and early 1970s, the full impact of technology and medical advancement was felt. In combination with the economic boom experienced by most countries at that time, this resulted in health care environments becoming bigger, more complex, more varied, more specialised and more sophisticated and, as a result of these trends, more costly. Concurrent with these changes was the demand by the health consumer for more and better quality health care. In accordance with these demands, medical aid and medical insurance schemes were established that enabled the health consumers, if they so wished and if they could afford these schemes, to have greater access to highly sophisticated specialised health care. As a result of these developments, private health care proliferated.

In accordance with the abovementioned changes and developments, the health team also became more complex and more specialised. Specialisation resulted in the expansion of the roles of the different members of the health team, with old roles becoming blurred and new roles emerging. As a result of these changes, new forms of education were required and new and more varied career patterns became available. At the same time, to meet the needs of specialisation and the greater demands for health care, new categories of health professionals emerged and supplementary and allied health professions were added to the health team. In South Africa, for example, the nursing team expanded to include not only the enrolled nurse and assistant nurse, but specialists in fields such as intensive care, theatre, anaesthetics, community health care and management.

This climate of specialisation was accompanied by the use of expensive, highly complex technology, with the result that increasing emphasis was given to the need for better management, higher productivity and more effective methods for measuring performance levels.

Consequently, during this period, health planning became more complex and more structured, but still remained mainly concerned with meeting only the needs of the health environment. These included both the needs of the health consumer and the health provider, with particular emphasis on the needs of highly specialised medical practitioners.

At this stage little attempt was made in health planning to set priorities or to coordinate or integrate health plans in a more comprehensive approach in a particular geographical or local area. Horizontal and vertical integration in the health planning process, if present, was found mainly in government health services and seldom expanded to include the non-health sector to any significant extent. In addition to this, health care institutions, services or programmes tended to function in isolation, catering for a specific need, with the total needs of the health consumer seldom being accommodated.

7.2.3 The health environment after 1975

The middle 1970s saw the beginning of the present economic recession experienced by most countries. Rising costs, diminishing resources, coupled with increasing demands for health care, necessitated that health planners should carefully examine the approaches used in the provision of health care as those currently in use were not only no longer cost effective, but no longer adequately met the total health needs of all the peoples they served.

The Alma Ata conference in 1978 heralded a new era for health environments. The changes that have taken place as a result of the recommendations made at that conference have had far-reaching implications for the planning of health care. Consequently, over the convening years, health care has evolved from a more curative institutional approach to the present health care environment in which the perspective is on health rather than on illness.

7.3 HEALTH AND HEALTH CARE IN SOUTH AFRICA

The philosophy and principles on which the primary health care approach is based are central to the approaches used for health and health care in South Africa. Health planning at all levels translates these principles into the mission, goals and objectives appropriate for implementation at a particular operational level.

According to Delport (1991:2), primary health care is regarded as:

> . . . essential health care based on scientifically sound and socially acceptable methods and technology made universally accessible to individuals and families in the community through their full participation and at a cost that the community and country can afford to maintain at every stage of their development in the spirit of self-reliance and self-determination. It forms an integral part both of South Africa's health systems, of which it is the central function and main focus, and of the overall social and economic development of the community. It is also the first level of contact of individuals, the family and the community with the national health system, bringing health care as close as possible to where the people live and work, and constitutes the first element of a continuing health care process.

7.4 PRIMARY HEALTH CARE CONCEPTS AND PRINCIPLES IMPORTANT IN HEALTH PLANNING

The implementation of the abovementioned definition of primary health care has required major changes in the attitudes of all the major role players in the health planning process. These developments have also had a major impact on the wider process of planning for health and health services.

7.4.1 Health concepts and primary health care

Health for planning purposes must be seen it its broadest context, i.e. as a state of complete physical, mental and social well-being.

Green (1994:49) maintains that health, viewed from this holistic perspective, can no longer be loosely interchanged with the terms health care, if health care is viewed purely from a medical perspective.

Health viewed in this wider context is affected by a number of factors, all of which must be considered in planning, as they can have a negative or positive impact on the total health of communities and individuals in a particular situation.

Figure 7.1 gives an outline of factors to be considered when planning for optimal levels of health and health care in an area.

This broader perception of health, which involves a wide section of society in the promotion of health, has required that in the planning process:

- communities and/or key role players should play a more pro-active role in their own health and that of others and that provision be made for this in the health planning process;
- greater attention be given to the perceived needs of the health care consumer and other health care providers;
- a more decentralised approach be used for health planning purposes;
- provision be made for greater community involvement and participation in decision-making throughout the health planning process; and
- provision be made for a "health-by-the-people" approach in the changes made for the future.

7.4.2 The accessibility principle and primary health care

In primary health care accessibility is defined as the continuing and organised supply of an equitable level of health care that is within easy reach of all citizens geographically, functionally, financially and culturally.

Geographical accessibility implies that the distance, travelling time and means of transport must be acceptable to the community served.

Financial accessibility implies that the services can be afforded by the community and the State.

Functional accessibility implies that the appropriate type of care is made available to those individuals who need it when necessary. This includes preventive, promotive, curative and rehabilitative health care. To incorp-

FIGURE 7.1 The components of a holistic definition of health

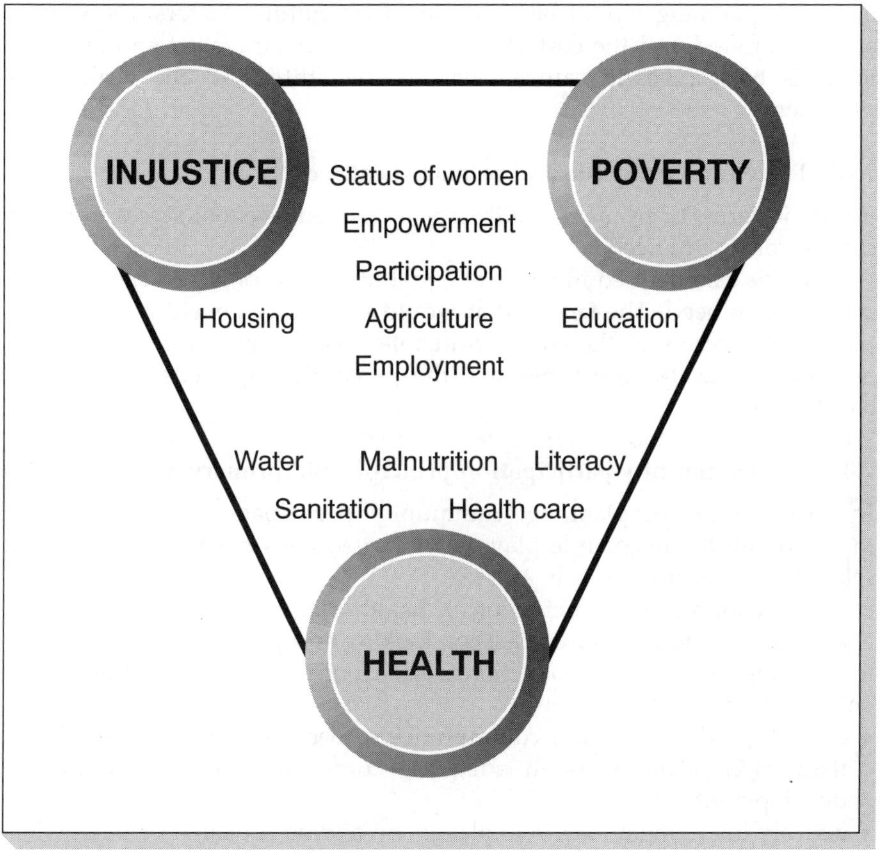

Source: Green (1994:23)

orate this into the health planning process, provision must be made for adequate referral systems.

7.4.3 The affordability principle and primary health care

Affordability in primary health care is defined as a level of health care that both the community and the health-care providers can afford.

Factors that would need to be considered in terms of this principle when planning for health or health care are fees charged, travel costs, the cost of drugs and lost income due to time spent away from work.

7.4.4 The acceptability principle and primary health care

Acceptability in terms of primary health care can be defined as a level of health or health care that is acceptable to the health care provider and health care consumer in terms of local needs and constraints. Acceptability in terms of health planning would be determined by cultural factors, the type of services offered and the cost of services, distances travelled and attitudes towards health, health care as well as the attitude of the health care providers.

7.4.5 The equity principle and primary health care

Equity in terms of primary health care is defined as equal access to health care, according to need.

Equity is also defined in terms of equal utilisation of health care services according to need. The factors that would need to be considered in health planning in terms of the equity principle relate to physical distance, the attitudes of health care providers, the perception of needs and cultural constraints.

7.4.6 The community participation principle and primary health care

In terms of health planning, community participation is enhanced by involving all the major role players when decisions have to be made that relate to health-care needs in an area.

Active community participation in health planning at operational level also results in more effective decision making and promotes a commitment to ensuring that the plans of action work. Community participation can be enhanced by:

- enabling individuals and communities to become more responsible for their own health through adequate communication, education and development;
- actively involving all key role players on a wide consultative basis when decisions have to be made in the health planning process; and
- promoting self-help schemes in the health planning process.

7.4.7 The appropriate technology principle and primary health care

In contemporary primary health care, emphasis is placed on technology that is appropriate to the local circumstances. Technology in this context refers to both equipment and material and also includes skilled personnel.

In deciding on the most appropriate resources for an area, the health planning team would need to consider the following:

- the needs, demands and constraints in an area;
- both capital and recurrent costs and whether these costs can be afforded by the community and/or the health care providers;
- factors that relate to efficiency and effectiveness in terms of local needs and the resources available;
- the acceptability of the resources to the community and to the health care providers; and

- the maintenance and replacement of buildings, equipment and materials at a local level.

7.4.8 The preventive promotive principle and primary health care

In meeting health needs, emphasis is currently being placed on promoting good health and preventing ill health. This principle is applied at primary, secondary and tertiary level. The health planning team, when planning a fully integrated coordinated comprehensive health care programme, needs to balance this principle with the needs for curative and rehabilitative health care.

In planning, the health planning team would need to make provision for:

- appropriate referral systems both horizontally and vertically;
- self-help approaches;
- a partnership relationship between government and the private sector;
- adequate support systems; and
- education and developmental programmes for all the major role players at operational level.

7.4.9 The decentralisation principle and primary health care

The delegation of decision-making power as close to the operational level as possible promotes a "bottom up" management approach and ensures more realistic planning. To accommodate this principle in the health planning process, provision should be made for:

- consultation on as wide a base as possible at operational level;
- the involvement of all the major role players on a regular basis at health-planning meetings; and
- adequate communication systems with regular feedback mechanisms between all the major role players.

7.5 FACTORS THAT PROMOTE SUCCESS IN HEALTH PLANNING

To be successful in promoting the health status of communities and individuals and to ensure health care that is appropriate to the needs and demands at operational level, health planning must incorporate clear procedures that:

- enable communities and health care providers to be involved on a regular basis when decisions have to be made related to health and health care needs;
- enable key role players from the health care sector as well as non-health sectors to be involved in health planning and decision-making; and
- facilitates the analysis and understanding of the various concepts, principles and terms used in the planning process and by so doing

makes the planning process democratic and transparent for the health care provider, the health care consumer and other sectors within the community.

7.5.1 What is health planning?

If the mission of "an optimum level of health care for all" is to be achieved, effective health planning on both a long- and short-term basis is of prime importance. Health planning, if it is to be effective, must be scientific and realistic in terms of local needs and resources. This can only be achieved if all the factors that could possibly affect the goals and objectives selected are identified, analysed, evaluated and monitored. Only then can programmes (plans of actions) remain viable in highly dynamic health environments and, at the same time, under today's stringent circumstances promote productivity, cost effectiveness and acceptance by the society they serve.

7.6 HEALTH PLANNING MODELS

Over the years, a number of health planning models have evolved in accordance with the various needs, philosophies and approaches used. Basically these models, when analysed, follow similar steps and are guided by similar principles. The planning approach selected should thus be one that is the most effective and appropriate for the specific circumstances required.

7.6.1 The epidemiological prevention process planning model

Clark (1992) uses the epidemiological prevention process model in planning for change in the health environment and identifies the steps in the planning process as assessment, diagnosis, planning, implementation and evaluation. Planning in this context is seen by Clarke (1992:193) as:

> . . . a continuous deliberate collaborative effort to improve the operation of a system. The planning process is seen as a series of tasks including establishing goals and objectives, evaluating alternative approaches to change, delineating activities that will lead to change and planning to evaluate change.

7.6.2 The problem-solving planning model

Clemen-Stone *et al.* (1991:423) regard health planning as

> . . . an ongoing process whereby information about a community is systematically collected and used to construct a usable plan. Health planning is seen as a problem-solving approach involving steps similar to those used in the nursing process.

In addition, there are the steps used in Clark's epidemiological prevention process model, i.e. pre-planning, assessment, policy development, implementation and evaluation.

Green (1994:23–24) regards planning as an explicit activity that attempts to determine how resources are used in relation to specific goals. He regards planning in this context as a series of steps as depicted in figure 7.2 below.

FIGURE 7.2: The mixed scanning cycle

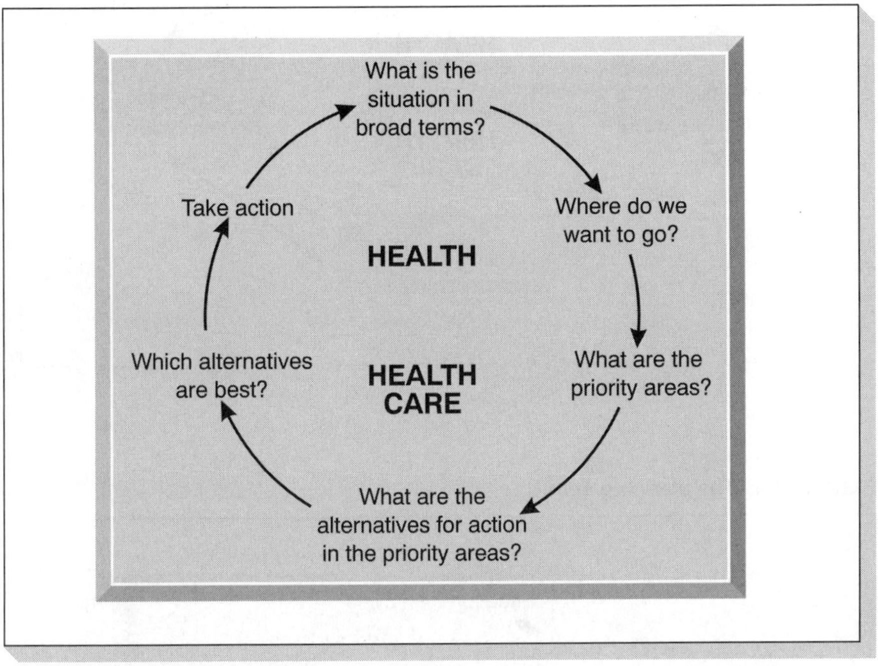

Source: Green (1994:25)

According to Green (1994:23), health planning can be divided into two levels, i.e.:

- *allocative planning:* deciding which activities are to be undertaken; and
- *activity planning:* setting time-tables or schedules for monitoring the implementation of plans.

As part of the health planning team, the community nurse is involved in planning activities at both these levels.

7.7 THE PLANNING PROCESS

Health planning incorporates the steps of assessment, planning, implementation and evaluation (see figure 7.3).

From a slightly different point of view, "health planning can also be seen as a planning spiral with the end points of each cycle forming the start of the next cycle, but at a higher plane" (Green 1994:31).

FIGURE 7.3: The four steps of health planning

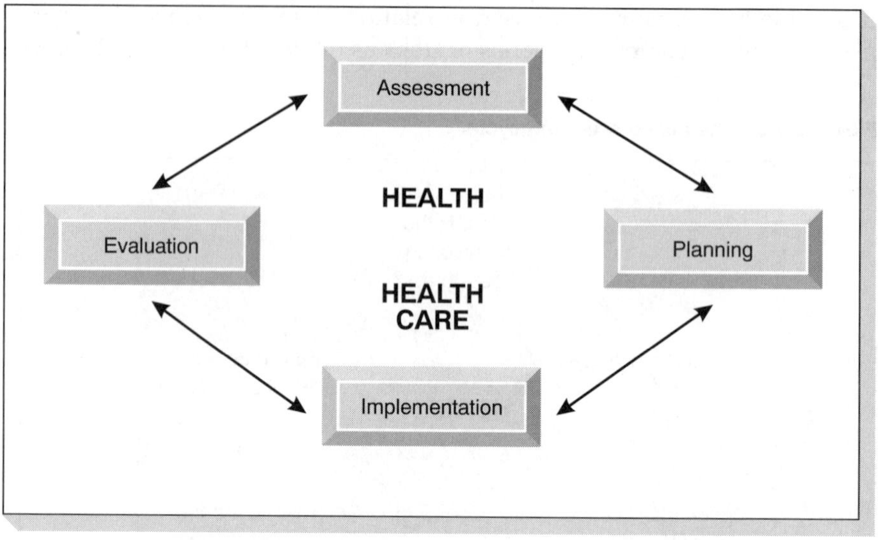

FIGURE 7.4: The planning spiral

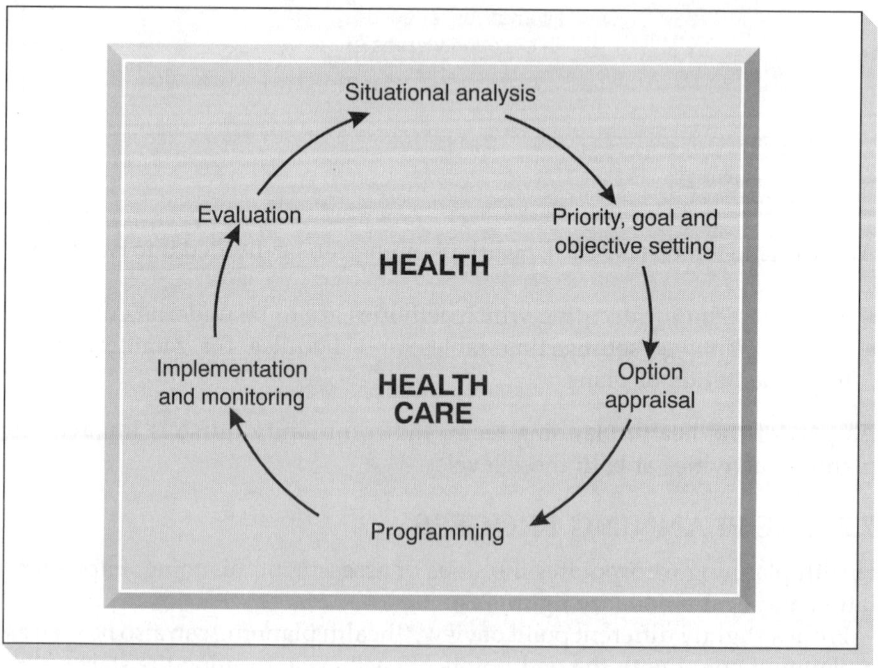

Source: Green (1994:31)

In terms of the two approaches outlined above, planning is regarded as a continuous process involving complex interrelated decisions that are taken simultaneously. The order in which the steps in the planning process are taken will, to a large extent, depend on the dynamics of the environment in which planning takes place.

7.7.1 Steps in the health-planning process

7.7.1.1 Situational analysis

As the first step in the planning process, assessment or situational analysis determines the nature of the situation on which health planning is focused. It is important to realise that the assessment process is a continuous one, especially in dynamic situations that can change dramatically, completely negating the initial assessment made. Assessment in health planning should focus on aspects such as the needs and demands for health care; the availability and suitability of current health facilities and programmes; manpower, material and financial resources; health, socio-economic, educational, demographic and political indicators, and the problems, issues, trends and developments present at both macro- and micro-levels. In assessing environments for health, it is essential that a market-orientated approach be used in which as wide a cross-section of the community is involved as possible. Only in this way will the information essential for realistic planning be obtained and will full commitment to health promotion and the concepts of primary health as essential health care at local level be promoted. The chapter on community assessment provides a detailed description of how a community assessment can be conducted.

7.7.1.2 Priority, goals and objective setting

Once full data about a particular environment have been collected, the data must be fully analysed to determine the most pressing needs and to identify the most significant problems. For decision-making purposes, the significance and/or implications of the data must be identified as, on the basis of this information, judgements can be made on which option will be the most feasible in terms of the goals to be met and the realities of the local circumstances.

7.8 THE COMPONENTS OF A HEALTH PROGRAMME AT PRIMARY HEALTH CARE LEVEL

In drawing up a health programme/project for implementation at operational level, the health planning team must clearly state the objectives of the health plan as well as the resources needed in terms of manpower, material and costs.

7.8.1 Objectives

The objectives of the health programme should clearly state what is to be done and when the tasks should be completed. The health-planning team should ensure that the objectives can be implemented. To achieve this:

- the necessary authority for implementation must be acquired;
- the necessary manpower, equipment, physical facilities, techniques and financial resources must be made available;
- laws and prevailing values and norms must be considered;
- the practical objectives must be attainable and relatively problem-free;
- the objectives must be acceptable to both the health-care providers and the health-care consumers; and
- the objectives should be measurable.

Once the objectives have been agreed upon, the specific tasks to be completed are detailed:

- *The objective:* What is to be done?
- *The manpower:* Who is responsible?
- *The location or facilities:* Where will the tasks be undertaken?
- *The resources:* What material resources, personnel, finances, buildings, transport, etc. are required?
- *The procedures policy:* How will the resources be used?
- *The time frame:* How long will it take to complete the tasks?

7.8.2 Manpower requirements

Manpower is a crucial element of planning strategies as the effectiveness of the programmes depends to a very large extent on the optimal utilisation of the full spectrum of manpower resources available. In relation to the procedure to be carried out and the services provided, the following information is needed:

- the number, category and grade of health nursing and non-health related personnel;
- the qualifications, level of experience and specific skills, together with the special equipment required;
- the availability of personnel and area of recruitment;
- the extent of training, support systems needed and additional facilities for training;
- the legal requirements and labour contracts, i.e. conditions of service and scope-of-practice regulations;
- salaries and fringe benefits;
- accommodation and transport needs;
- staff norms and expectations;
- constraints in terms of manpower provision; and
- cost implications.

7.8.3 Material resources

The factors to consider when planning for material resources are equipment, supplies and the building or space needed to carry out the tasks identified. In addition to this, the required support systems should be identified, i.e. linen, laundry, catering, transport, pharmaceutical supplies, stores, general maintenance and any other additional services in the community. Questions to be asked in this regard relate to how the required resource would be requisitioned, stored, distributed, repaired, replaced, monitored and controlled, funded and costed at operational level.

7.8.4 Budgeting

A major aspect in health planning is to determine the costs associated with each item, or the procedures of the proposed health plan or programme. Detailed costing of each item and each activity is required for both capital and recurrent costs in terms of buildings, equipment, supplies and manpower. All these factors need to be considered by the health-planning team when deciding on the most appropriate option for implementing health plans.

7.8.5 Option appraisal

In selecting the most appropriate goals and objectives for meeting health and health-care needs at operational level, it is important to realise that in planning, change is inevitable. Change has a ripple effect, therefore the implications of change throughout the system in which health planning is taking place must be assessed, as a strategy or programme considered ideal for the health system may, for example, not be the most optimal in terms of the total needs of the community. It is for this reason that alternative options must be devised and that it is necessary that these options should be carefully evaluated and judged in accordance with specific criteria. The criteria drawn up must be accepted and understood by the entire health-planning team. This requires a problem-solving approach in which the strengths, weaknesses, opportunities and threats inherent in a particular situation are identified, analysed and fully discussed. To be fully effective, each option must be broken down into its component parts in terms of the policies, procedures, manpower, material resources, time and money needed. Each item can then be judged by each member of the health-planning team by measuring it against the predetermined criteria.

The predetermined criteria used to select the optimal option for implementation in a particular situation are those that promote:

- health and the quality of health care;
- cost-effectiveness and productivity; and
- high staff morale.

Each option can be judged or measured against the extent to which each is accessible, affordable, cost-effective, acceptable and meets the equity principle under the local circumstances.

7.8.6 Cost benefit analysis

A cost benefit analysis is one method often used in determining the most appropriate option to be selected. In this method, strategies are drawn up in detail and the consequences of each alternative approach to be used are predicted, costed over a period of time and compared. De Bella *et al.* (1986:33) maintain that

> . . . cost benefit analysis is useful as it forces health planners to examine alternative choices in the context of limited resources and that with competing possibilities, the selection must be based on efficient allocation of resources.

The other important advantage of a cost benefit analysis is that it integrates the planning and budgeting process, thus enabling options to relate more easily to the financial realities of a situation. A cost benefit analysis also enables health planners to become more innovative and creative, as it requires the strength and opportunities identified in a situation to be combined and, where possible, the weaknesses and threats eliminated or reduced.

7.8.7 Criteria-weighting techniques

Another method that can be used in selecting appropriate options is one in which cost-utility comparisons can be made in non-currency terms. In this method, the consideration of efficiency and effectiveness is based on the rating scales and values of the health-planning team. It is important that the health-planning team should be drawn from a wide range of disciplines, as different views, descriptions, perspectives and experiences are needed in the decision-making process.

In this method, weightings are assigned to criteria and to the options to be used, indicating the value of each. Significant levels are then determined for prioritising purposes. Numbers are assigned to each criterion by using a scale, for example, from one to five. Individual members of the health-planning team are then required to rate the importance of each criterion by allocating it a number from this scale. The numbers allocated by individual members of the health-planning team are then totalled and averaged, resulting in a single value being allocated to each criterion. This number indicates the relative importance given to the criterion by the health-planning team.

Initially, individual members of the health-planning team rate the importance of the alternative options to be used against the criteria drawn up. They are required to select a score from a range of numbers, for example from minus 10 to plus 10. The individual rating score of each member of the health-planning team is then totalled and averaged, resulting in a single plus or minus number. This number reflects the consensus of the health-planning team in relation to the value for a particular option.

Significance levels are obtained by multiplying the weighting given to each criterion by the rating given for each option. All the significant levels for each option are then totalled so that a composite value is obtained for all the criteria. This single number reflects the view of the health-planning team on the relative usefulness of each option.

7.8.8 Programming

Once the preferred option has been selected, the plan of action is costed and detailed, indicating who will do what, where, when and how.

7.8.9 Implementation and monitoring

Once the programme/plan has been selected, it is necessary to ensure that the plan of action will be effectively implemented at operational level. This requires commitment at operational level, which can be obtained by:

- clearly stating who does what, where, when and how;
- appointing an individual responsible for coordinating the whole programme at operational level and for ensuring that the tasks are carried out on time;
- ensuring that all the materials and equipment are available and that the staff involved have been briefed and trained for the changes taking place;
- listing steps in order of sequence and identifying completion dates for the tasks;
- consulting those involved to identify potential problem areas; and
- specifying the resources needed and possible problems.

A technique commonly used, which is discussed in detail in most planning books for monitoring the implementation of a planning strategy, is the programme evaluation and review technique (PERT). PERT permits planners to develop a map for the plotting activities to be carried out and records results in a network diagram that depicts the total flow of events. The diagram can be designed in such a way that additional steps can be added. PERT also permits an evaluation and necessary adjustments to the strategy, so that objectives can be completed on time.

Figure 4 gives an example of the time-monitoring schedule that can be used at operational level for the implementation of a health programme.

An example of a critical path analysis is given in Figure 7.6 below. It shows an analysis of the time taken to carry out the various activities involved in the construction of a basic building. The shortest time for completion is 51 days, which is calculated as the sum of the foundation (10 days), walls (20 days), electrical (10 days), electrical checks (one day) and painting (10 days).

FIGURE 7.5: Bar chart for the implementation of a health-care project

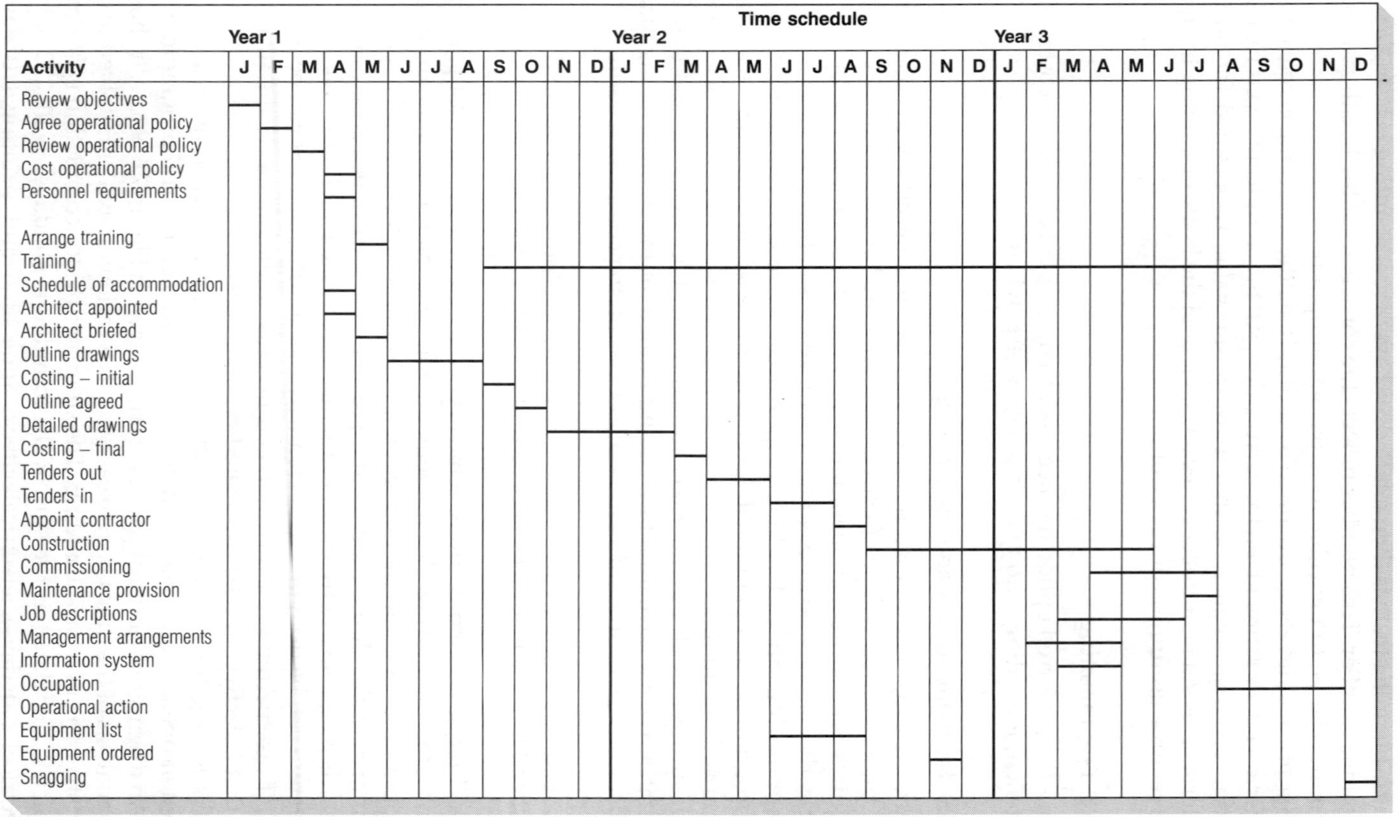

Source: Green (1994:284)

A delay in any of the critical events would lead to an overall delay in completion. The other activities of roofing and plumbing have some slack time. Some delay in these events would not delay the overall completion date.

FIGURE 7.6: A critical path analysis

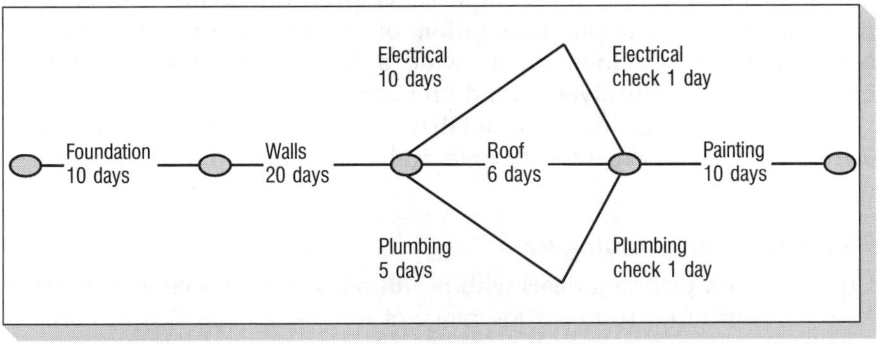

Source: Green (1994:285)

7.8.10 Evaluation

Evaluation in the health planning process is much more than just a feedback mechanism. It must be seen as a continuous integral part of the total planning process. Evaluation is needed to assess the outcome and effectiveness of the health programmes. It is also needed to control operations in terms of the activities carried out and the money spent. Evaluation can also form the basis and provide incentives for further health planning and change.

Basically, evaluation is done to ensure that the quality of the services is maintained, productivity is enhanced and health objectives are met.

Evaluation means that the predetermined criteria, standards, norms and objectives must be identified against which the activities and progress can be measured. It is also necessary to indicate who will be responsible for monitoring the programme and how frequently this should take place.

Different methods such as management by objective and programme budgeting can be used to evaluate the effectiveness of the procedures and health programmes. The methods used are determined by the purpose of the evaluation and the criteria, norms and standards agreed upon.

Information for evaluation purposes can be obtained:

- through performance appraisal of health care providers;
- through surveys and research projects;
- from health reports, health records, health statistics and health indicators;
- through direct observation;
- from attendance records;
- from feedback given at meetings;

- from individuals through direct contact or through questionnaires; and
- through audits.

7.9 THE COMMUNITY NURSE AS A MEMBER OF THE HEALTH PLANNING TEAM

To accommodate and facilitate the changes taking place in the health care environment in South Africa, emphasis is given to decentralisation, open lines of communication, integration of services both vertically and horizontally, consultation on as wide a base as possible, community involvement, cost effectiveness and productivity.

In health planning, this has meant that the approaches used should be pro-active, innovative, creative, flexible and permit maximum input at the operational level.

7.9.1 The health planning team

Current health planning deals with health-related and social issues and as such requires input from a wide range of interest groups that include the health-care consumer, health professionals from various disciplines, the private sector and non-governmental organisations as well as specialists in health planning. If buildings are involved, architects are also required.

The community nurse has a major role to play in these health-planning teams as she is in a central position at primary health-care level and is also in a unique position, as she is in continuous direct contact with the community. This, combined with her knowledge of the needs and problems in her area, enables her closely to monitor the changes taking place. A knowledge of these changes, combined with her experience and her knowledge of future developments, enables her to hold a position in the health-planning team where she can make valuable contributions to the discussions held and the ultimate decisions made in relation to the most appropriate options for health and health care in her region.

The contributions the community nurse makes to the decisions taken by the health-planning team can only remain effective if she is continually alert to all the facets of change in her immediate environment, as well as to the changes taking place at macro-level that could directly or indirectly affect health and health care in her region or that could have implications for health planning.

The information that the community nurse obtains in relation to the changes in the community she serves should be current, accurate and represent the views of the different groups, disciplines, community leaders, consumers of health care, providers of health care and relevant health and nursing teams. This will only be possible if networking systems are established at local level, in which there are open lines of communication, full consultation and contact on a regular basis in a climate of mutual trust and respect.

A climate of mutual trust and respect will only be established if the community nurse is visible and regarded as knowledgeable and competent and is able to communicate effectively in a group context.

In assessing the worth of the information obtained for health-planning purposes, the community nurse must:

- be fully conversant with the current mission, goals, health programmes, policies procedures and laws operative at macro- and micro-level;
- be sensitive to changing needs and the needs of the other members of the health planning team;
- recognise and understand the impact of change both now and in the future on the total environment;
- be future-orientated;
- be assertive and confident in the health planning team and present the information in a concise, logical and systematic format; and
- develop the ability to integrate present and future plans into integrated, coordinated and comprehensive health-care approaches.

7.10 SUMMARY

Purposeful health planning is essential if the overall mission of an optimal level of health for all the people in South Africa is ultimately to be achieved. The health programmes or projects selected must be feasible in terms of present and future health and health-care needs. The decisions made should be based on a comprehensive knowledge of the total environment as well as the consensus of the health planning team, which is representative of all the major role players at operational level.

Health-planning approaches must be flexible, innovative and creative. The approaches used should facilitate the need for rapid change, cost effectiveness, productivity, quality care and commitment. Effective health planning in this context should:

- be pro-active and future-orientated;
- be realistic and feasible for local circumstances;
- use a total approach involving both the health and the non-health sector;
- involve a wide spectrum of interest groups, both at a horizontal and a vertical level;
- promote intersectoral, interdisciplinary and community participation and commitment through open lines of communication networking and consultation in the form of health forums, tasks groups, etc;
- facilitate critical analytical thought and informed decision-making on a broad and, where possible, a scientific base; and
- allow for contingency planning.

QUESTIONS

1. Define planning and indicate the basic requirements of health planners for effective planning.

2. Briefly discuss the changes that have taken place in health environments since the beginning of the twentieth century and indicate the impact these changes have had on health and health care.
3. List and briefly discuss the different planning approaches that can be used in health care planning.
4. Identify planning principles considered important in the health planning process
5. In planning a particular health care programme/service, a number of options are available in terms of the planning strategies to be used. Briefly discuss the methods that can be used to assist you in selecting the most appropriate strategy.
6. Discuss the importance of objectives in health programmes.
7. In planning health programmes, resources are required to achieve the objectives set. Identify these resources and discuss the factors you would need to consider to ensure that the resources provided are appropriate.
8. A health programme is to be implemented in your area. How would you ensure that the health care plan is successfully implemented.
9. Evaluation is an integral part of the health planning process. Discuss this statement.
10. The community nurse has a vital part to play in health planning for her region (area). Defend this statement.

FURTHER READING

The relevant chapters on health planning in Clark, M.J. 1996. *Nursing in the community.* 2nd edition. Norwalk, Connecticut: Appleton & Lange.

Green, A. 1994. *An introduction to health planning in developing countries.* Oxford: Oxford University Press.

WHO publications and any contemporary article in relevant journals on health planning.

BIBLIOGRAPHY

Clark, M.J. 1992. *Nursing in the community.* Norwalk, Connecticut: Appleton & Lange.

Clemen-Stone, S., Eigiste, D. & McGuire, S.L. 1991. *Comprehensive family and community health nursing.* 3rd edition. St Louis: Mosby.

De Bella, S., Martin, S. & Siddal, S. 1986. *Nurses' role in health care planning.* Norwalk, Connecticut: Appleton & Lange.

Delport, A. 1991. *Strategy for primary health care in South Africa.* Pretoria: Department of National Health and Population Development.

Green, A. 1994. *An introduction to health planning in developing countries.* Oxford: Oxford University Press.

8 Indicators to monitor progress towards the attainment of the goal of health for all by the year 2000

MARIE DREYER

CHAPTER OBJECTIVES

After reading this chapter, the student should be able to:

- define the term "indicator";
- outline the various indicators to monitor progress;
- describe what is meant by "health for all"; and
- apply the indicators to evaluate the health status of South Africa.

8.1 INTRODUCTION

With the declaration of Alma Ata in 1978 the concept of primary health care as the key to improving the health status and the quality of life of all people in the world was accepted. According to the World Health Organisation (1981:3):

> Alma Ata is a name that has become synonymous with one of the great public health movements of history, namely the quest for equity in health, expressed as WHO's goal of Health for All by the year 2000.

"Health for all by the year 2000" does not mean that there will be no sickness or disability, or that sufficient health manpower will be available. It means that health personnel will have to teach people to take responsibility for their own health and health-care delivery as well as for the health of their families. It means that people will become aware of the fact that certain diseases can be prevented and that life-styles can be changed to improve health. It also means that essential health-care services will be evenly distributed and accessible to all individuals and families in an acceptable and affordable way and with their full participation (WHO 1981:79–85).

Since the acceptance of the Alma Ata declaration, countries have been motivated to show increased commitment to introducing essential primary health care and developing infrastructures that meet the health-care needs of their people. In this regard, in 1981, the World Health Assembly invited member states to implement strategies, to monitor the progress towards the attainment of the goal of health for all and to evaluate the effectiveness of this goal by using appropriate indicators. Uniform criteria to prove commitment and to measure what has been accomplished were introduced by the World Health Organisation. It has also been recommended that progress should be regularly monitored and that effectiveness should be evaluated every second year.

8.2 A DEFINITION OF THE TERM "INDICATOR"

The World Health Organisation defines indicators as "variables which help to measure changes" (WHO 1981:12). Indicators thus give an indication or a reflection of a certain situation and are sometimes used when changes cannot be directly measured. Indicators should, for example, be valid. In other words, they should measure what they are supposed to measure. They must also be objective, sensitive and specific. In reality few indicators comply with all these criteria.

Indicators can also be used as yardsticks to compare the progress of one country with another, especially in the case of countries with similar levels of socio-economic development. In this chapter the focus will fall mainly on the situation in South Africa but some international comparison will be included where applicable.

Since health may mean many different things to different people, indicators are necessary to illustrate to individuals whether they are making progress. Indicators are also useful to monitor health care programmes at different levels, such as national, local or district level. The usefulness of an indicator may be determined by the organisational, technical and financial feasibility of the collection and analysis of required data (WHO 1981:12–14). Indicators are also essential in the planning of health services.

8.3 CATEGORIES OF INDICATORS TO MONITOR PROGRESS

Four categories of indicators were recommended by the World Health Organisation (WHO 1981).

8.3.1 Health policy indicators

Health policy includes aspects such as political commitment to the goal of optimal health for all, resource allocation, the degree of equity of distribution of health resources, community involvement in attaining optimal health for all, and an organisational framework and managerial process.

8.3.1.1 Political commitment

The World Health Organisation sees political commitment as an essential element in the achievement of the goal "health for all". Indicators of political commitment are especially important in the early stages to evaluate the extent of commitment of a country. These indicators are largely qualitative and include aspects such as the allocation of financial resources, the degree of community involvement and the establishment of a suitable organisational framework. Political commitment to reduce socio-economic disparities and to provide essential health care services and facilities is essential if the goal of health for all is to be achieved.

South Africa has also accepted the primary health-care approach and committed itself to bringing health services to all the inhabitants of the country. The 1994 National Health Plan of the ANC clearly indicates that health-care delivery in South Africa will be based on the primary health-care approach and that the government is committed to promoting social and economic development. Endeavours are thus made to follow the guidelines of the World Health Organisation. The philosophy for primary health care in South Africa is based on the principles of partnership between the private sector and health authorities, as well as community involvement and liaison with local communities (South Africa (b) 1991). In 1996 the Department of Health decided that the primary health-care approach should take precedence in all health matters with the emphasis on prevention and that the new health system should be based on:

- decentralisation without fragmentation;
- a comprehensive package;
- equity; and
- intersectoral collaboration.

It was decided that the District Health System would be the cornerstone of health-care delivery in South Africa .

To be able to meet the goal of primary health care and to improve the quality of life of all people, certain priority areas and target groups were identified:

- provision for basic needs, such as water, housing, sewage and refuse removal, and provision of adequate food;
- health education;
- attention to self-help, community development and participation;
- promotion of the health of certain vulnerable groups such as mothers and children, women, workers, the aged and victims of violence;
- decentralisation of health services to make these services more accessible at grassroots level; and
- provision of essential medicine to treat patients in clinics, etc.

8.3.1.2 Financial resource allocation

It is essential that equitable resource allocation, *per capita* expenditure, as well as human resources, technology and facilities for primary health care should be available to all population groups and within geographical areas (WHO 1981:40).

Financial resource allocation refers to the amount of money made available in the annual budget for various purposes, for example health care, housing, environmental services, employment, food production, education, etc.

The health budget, according to the World Health Organisation (1981) is of special importance in a country's commitment towards health for all. The specific amount of money allocated for health, as well as that available for the provision of primary health care, should be clearly defined. The allocation of funds is based on the proportion of the gross national product available for health services. Equally important is the pattern indicated of actual distribution to areas where there is a definite need, for example to people who do not have reasonable access to primary health care, clean water, proper housing and other essential services and facilities (WHO 1981:21–22).

The World Health Organisation has set a target that at least five per cent of the GNP should be spent on health by all countries, and a reasonable percentage of this should be spent on primary health care. In 1992/1993 South Africa spent 5,4% on health care in comparison with 2 to 3% in developing countries and 5 to 10% in developed countries. According to a World Health Organisation Report (1995), some developing countries spent less than 1% of the GNP on health.

8.3.1.3 Community involvement and participation

Community involvement in health care is recognised all over the world as one of the basic requirements for attaining the goal of health for all by the year 2000. Community involvement refers to the process whereby communities, families and individuals assume responsibility for their own health and welfare and develop the capacity to contribute to their own development and to that of the community (WHO 1995:225).

The degree to which the community is involved in decision-making and active participation in health matters, is seen as a major indication of the seriousness of the political commitment of a specific government to this concept. People should be encouraged to become actively involved in decision making and to take responsibility for some of the decisions made on health-related matters, especially at local level. The importance of the involvement of the community in health-care provision cannot be overemphasised. Community members have a right as well as a duty to participate in health-care delivery and the development of health-care services.

The extent of community involvement can be related to the progress made in the decentralisation of health care and the co-operation and partnership between the providers of health care and the community at that level.

To maintain a satisfactory level of health, active and continued participation by individuals in the community is required. The attitudes, habits and behaviour of the individual, the family or the community can either promote or undermine health concepts and health care.

All regions of the World Health Organisation find community involvement important for developing primary health care as well as for becoming self-reliant. Active participation is a tool to empower communities to make their own decisions regarding the development of health-care facilities and other needs.

In South Africa, community involvement and active participation are emphasised and encouraged. Health promotion and health maintenance enjoy high priority and people are encouraged to take responsibility for their own health and well-being by means of their own resources combined with outside support. Intersectoral collaboration is closely related to and encouraged in community development to bring various communities and sectors of communities with appropriate knowledge and expertise together to facilitate the process of community development and participation.

8.3.1.4 Organisational framework and managerial process

A national managerial process is required to ensure that the principles of primary health care are implemented. A sound philosophy and policy should be adopted in this regard and strategies and mechanisms should be developed to implement the policy of primary health care in a specific country.

The effectiveness of the organisation of the national health care system of a country can serve as an indicator of political commitment. Factors to consider are effective communication, the involvement of medical and nursing schools and other organisations in research related to primary health care, the development of district health committees, the integration of primary, secondary and tertiary health care, as well as the co-ordination and integration of health services and the development of suitable strategies to provide health care.

Although most countries claim that they have developed national health policies and strategies to provide health care for all people, problems still exist in terms of effective implementation because of a lack of legislative support and resources. The World Health Organisation reported in 1987 that conflicting national targets made progress very difficult and the lack of skilled managers at local level often hampers decentralisation and the development of district- and community-based health-care services.

During the period from 1980 to 1986, the effectiveness of the health services in South Africa was investigated and certain problem areas were identified. Similar to the findings in many other countries, the shortage of money, shortage of human resources, unequal distribution of health-care services as well as human resources were some of the problem areas identified.

To ensure South Africa's commitment to rendering primary health care services to all its inhabitants, primary health care was further expanded and provision has been made for strategies to combat measles and diarrhoea-related diseases in children. Immunisation programmes were also expanded, more community health centres were erected, and mobile units were purchased (South Africa (b) 1991) and decentralised to operational level. These improvements are now seen as essential comprehensive health-care delivery at local level.

In the new national health plan for South Africa (ANC:1994) great emphasis is placed on the development, reorientation and redistribution of human resources as well as the development of physical infrastructures for health-care delivery to be able to reach all people.

8.3.2 Social and economic indicators

Social and economic indicators do not directly measure the progress made towards the attainment of the goal of health for all, but are closely related to the influences from outside that affect health. These indicators, because of their direct impact on health, are seen as being of great importance in the interpretation of health status and in the provision of health services. These indicators include demographic factors such as age, sex distribution, population growth and urbanisation. Economic indicators include factors such as gross national product, income distribution, employment/unemployment levels, adult literacy, housing and the availability of food.

Health personnel world-wide would agree that there is a close relationship between population growth, socio-economic development and the health status of individuals. The fast-growing populations are among the main problems in the world and are also a major constraint in reaching the goal of health for all.

Social welfare includes the right to meet basic needs such as shelter, food, health care, work opportunities, income security and other factors that can promote the physical, social and emotional well-being of all people in a society.

8.3.2.1 Gross national product (GNP)

The gross national product as an indicator relates to the size of the national economy. It serves as a measure of change in the total output from which a share must go to the provision of health care. It can also serve as a measure of human welfare (WHO:1981). The *per capita* income of a country will have an influence on its health status as well as on the quality of life of its inhabitants. But of even greater importance are the nature and level of economic development attained in a country. It should be realised, however, that even the richest countries cannot always provide the best health care for even their wealthiest people. In this regard, some countries with a high GNP have the health status of third-world countries. The economic policy of a country considerably influences the health-care policy, as well as the priorities and objectives related to health-care programmes. In the evaluation of the health performance of a country, the two most important factors considered are the general developmental stages of the community and their general level of affluence. Planners world-wide also realise that improvements in the health status of a country have a positive influence on social and economic development in general.

If countries are to provide for basic needs such as work, food, housing and water, an annual economic growth of at least 6% for developing countries is recommended by the World Health Organisation. In many of these countries the economic growth per annum is estimated at only 2,5%, thus the basic needs are not being met for large portions of the population. According to the WHO (1995:181), in the least developed countries the average GNP grew at an average rate of 1–5% in the last decade. However, according to this report, the population growth is a great constraint and outstripped or was equal to the economic growth. In some countries that are in economic transition, the economic rates ranged from 0,5–4% while in developed countries they ranged from 1–4,3%.

South Africa is classified as a middle-income country by the World Bank but there has been a decline in the economy over the past decade with a negative growth rate in 1991 and 1992. In 1994 the growth rate increased to 2,5% but further growth is necessary to reduce unemployment (Department of Health 1995:17).

*8.3.2.2 **Adult literacy***

According to the World Health Organisation, the recommended literacy rate for both adult men and women should exceed 70% of the total population. The literacy rate in this context is seen as the percentage of a population, aged 15 and over, able to read and write in any language (WHO 1981:24). The literacy level of women is regarded as being of great importance in the provision of primary health care. Women who are literate can be trained and utilised as primary health-care workers, and are also able to understand and interpret health-education programmes. Their involvement will have an important influence on the health status of children as well as the rest of the community. Research has shown that child health and infant mortality can be related to the literacy of mothers.

The literacy rate in some developing countries is still very low. Some African countries have a literacy rate of between 20 to 40%, in comparison with South Africa, where the literacy rate is between 60 and 70%. According to UNESCO, as cited by the WHO (1995:181), the literacy level of women lags behind in most developing regions and in some of these regions it is reported to be only half that of men because of educational discrimination against girls.

*8.3.2.3 **Housing***

This indicator reflects the adequacy of housing in a community, including the number of persons per room, the nature of accommodation, size, insulation against extremes in weather conditions, the exclusion of rodents and disease-carrying insects, as well as ventilation, water provision and sanitation. Housing may have a direct influence on the physical and mental health of a population as well as on its social well-being.

Housing is a factor that may influence the quality of life of people and socio-economic development has a great impact on housing and well-being. In developing rural areas as well as in overpopulated urban areas housing is often inadequate and of poor quality, which results in health and health-related problems such as alcoholism, violence, teenage pregnancies, etc.

8.3.2.4 Working conditions

Indicators on working conditions reflect the employment/unemployment rate of a country as well as the economic dependency rate. They also give an indication of the percentage of women in the labour force, as well as the prevalence of disability preventing gainful employment. The dependency rate is seen as the number of persons under the age of 15 years and those aged 65 or older per 1 000 persons between the ages of 15 and 64 (WHO 1981:24).

The employment/unemployment rate has a definite influence on the economic circumstances and the quality of life of individuals. In developing countries, health problems are largely related to poverty, which results in insufficient food, overcrowded houses and a lack of sanitation facilities. Poverty is a critical factor in health-care planning in developing countries and is a predominant cause of poor health.

In South Africa 57% of the total population falls within the 15-to-64-year category (Development Bank 1991). South Africa has a low labour absorbtion capacity and about 40% of the economically active population of South Africa is unemployed. Women are disproportionately poorly represented in the labour market.

8.3.3 Indicators of the provision of primary health care

Currently there are no satisfactory indicators for the provision of health care or health-care coverage. Consequently, indicators generally accepted to measure these aspects are those covered by terms such as availability, accessibility, utilisation of services and quality of health care. According to the World Health Organisation, the progress in the implementation of primary health care could be measured in terms of the degree to which the health status has changed.

8.3.3.1 Accessibility

The term "accessibility" is defined as the number or portion of a given population that can be expected to use a specific facility or service, with the assumption that certain barriers can exist (WHO 1981:27). Accessibility can be broken down into the following components:

- *Physical accessibility:* This may have a different meaning in different countries, for example in some countries it may mean within one hour's walking distance, while in another it may be half an hour's travel by ox-cart. It is therefore necessary to define physical accessibility in terms of objectives for each of the elements of primary health care. According to the World Health Organisation (1981:27), coverage can be assessed by measuring the proportion of the population within an acceptable distance from the essential services in the different geographical or administrative areas. Physical access may also relate to the referral facilities.
- *Economic accessibility:* This refers to an individual's ability to meet the cost of the available health care. If health care is not affordable, it is not accessible.
- *Cultural accessibility:* This refers to the acceptability of services provided to the community. Acceptability in this context implies that the services must be relevant to the needs of the people to whom they are provided.

*8.3.3.2 **Utilisation of services***

The utilisation of services can be influenced by factors such as accessibility, affordability, quality of care and lack of essential medicine. The coverage of the population through available services can be expressed as the number of people in need of a service who actually receive the required service; for example the proportion of children at risk who are immunised. It is necessary that each country should specify the minimum standards of care that must be attained to ensure proper coverage. The number of people who actually use a service can be obtained through proper recording systems.

*8.3.3.3 **Quality of care***

Health care is very complex and to evaluate the results of the health-care process is thus extremely difficult. Various processes can contribute to the improvement of the health status of a community, such as social indicators, as well as cultural, political and economic conditions. A number of indicators are therefore required to measure the quality of health care provided. These can be built into monitoring systems by using check-lists and/or a scoring system. In addition to this, regular supervision and inspections are necessary to ensure that high standards of health care are attained and maintained, especially in rural areas. Quality assurance programmes should involve evaluation as well as improvement activities. To be effective, the criteria and standards for these programmes must be clearly defined. The extent to which services are utilised can be an indication of the quality of care provided. Quality control, however, requires far more complex indicators.

*8.3.3.4 **Primary health care coverage***

Primary health care coverage is only really meaningful, according to the World Health Organisation (1981:28), when it relates to the services that the national strategy of a country aims at providing. Indicators to measure the extent of primary health care coverage relate to the following critical elements of primary health care:

- health literacy;
- information and education concerning health to promote health literacy;
- the nature and extent of food supply and the improvement of the nutritional status;
- the degree of accessibility to water and sanitation facilities;
- the accessibility to maternity and child health care, including family planning;
- the percentage of children at risk immunised against the major infectious diseases;
- the prevention and control of endemic diseases;
- the appropriate treatment of common diseases and injuries;
- the provision of essential drugs;
- coverage by the referral system; and
- the ratio of population to available health manpower and the rural/urban distribution.

According to the World Health Organisation (1995), many countries report considerable progress in terms of delivery of primary health care. Developed countries have reported an 80 to 100% coverage with some essential elements of primary health care, while in developing countries access is still inequitable, particularly in rural and poor urban areas.

Although improvements are made in providing water and basic sanitation facilities, the growing problem of squatter and slum areas in some cities is working against the provision of primary health care and the situation can deteriorate despite all the efforts being made by these countries. The accessibility of essential services and facilities such as health care, water and sanitation is hampered by uncontrolled urbanisation and the settlement of large numbers of people where no services exist or where the available services are insufficient. Communities in informal settlements always suffer from a lack of health infrastructures, and consequently from malnutrition and other diseases related to poor socio-economic conditions (Development Bank 1991:22–23).

According to the World Health Organisation, 25 000 people still die every day of water-borne diseases such as cholera and gastro-enteritis because of insufficient sanitation facilities and poor drinking-water supplies.

The World Health Organisation (1995) also reports that immunisation is receiving high priority in most countries, and that countries such as Brazil, Sri Lanka and others have made impressive improvement. Progress has also been made in the availability of appropriate treatment for common diseases and injuries as well as in the availability of essential drugs at first level.

The South African health authorities also place special emphasis on the essential elements recommended by the World Health Organisation and focus on good quality primary health care that is accessible, affordable and acceptable to all the people of the country. The maintenance of personal health, self-medication, healthy life-styles, fitness and correct nutrition are emphasised in health education programmes (Delport 1991).

8.3.4 Basic health status indicators

Certain specific indicators were identified by the World Health Organisation to evaluate the health status of the inhabitants of a country. They are, among others, the nutritional status of children, infant mortality, child mortality, life expectancy at a given age, maternal mortality, disease-specific mortality and morbidity. Mortality data form the basis for assessing the health status of populations and the infant mortality rate is considered an accurate indicator for assessing the health status of children.

According to the World Health Organisation (1987:113) ". . . the ultimate impact of the health-for-all strategy must be measured by the improvement in the health status of the population".

8.3.4.1 Nutritional status

The nutritional status is a positive health indicator because of the availability of measurements to assess the growth and development of young children. Birth weight is an important indicator of a community's nutritional level. Weight-for-age is the most commonly used measure of the nutritional status. Weight-for-height is used to measure the current nutritional status and can give an indication of the extent to which a person is acutely malnourished. The growth of a child is related to the nutrition of the child and therefore measurement of growth is one of the indicators of nutritional status. Nutrition has a direct impact on infant and child survival. Training and education are essential for nutritional improvement, and supplementary feeding programmes can be implemented as direct measures for providing the most deprived population groups with additional food.

The World Health Organisation indicates that at least 90% of newborn infants should have a birth weight of 2 500 g and that 90% of children must have a weight that corresponds to the recommended weight-for-age.

Growth and development are shown by an increase in weight and height. Nutrition surveys look at the height and weight of a child in relation to age and to weight-for-height to get a picture of the nutritional status of children in a specific community (Byrne & Bennett 1986:82).

8.3.4.2 Psychosocial development

The psychosocial development of children is as important as their physical growth and development. These indicators should be determined within the specific community as they are influenced by the culture of the community concerned. The first year of development is very important because the child grows rapidly physically, mentally, emotionally and socially. Malnutrition can retard the whole process of growth and development of a child and correct nutrition from before birth is therefore essential.

8.3.4.3 *Infant mortality*

The infant mortality rate has always been recognised as one of the most important indicators of the health status of a population. Unreliable notification and statistics are, however, a huge obstacle in some developing countries, and it is an almost impossible task to obtain reliable figures in this regard.

Child mortality and the prevalence of communicable diseases are regarded as reliable indicators of standards of hygiene, nutrition and life-style, as well as of the level of preventative and promotive health care of a population.

The World Health Organisation recommends an infant mortality rate of below 50 per 1 000 live births as acceptable. In some developing countries the infant mortality rate is still as high as 200 per 1 000 live births, while in developed countries it is only 15 per 1 000 live births. A large variation can also exist within the same country, for instance between rural and urban areas or between population groups with different socio-economic levels (WHO 1981:34).

Factors influencing infant mortality are:
- the general nutritional status;
- available antenatal and maternity services;
- the educational standard of mothers;

FIGURE 8.1: Infant mortality rate for South Africa in 1994 (per 1 000 live births)

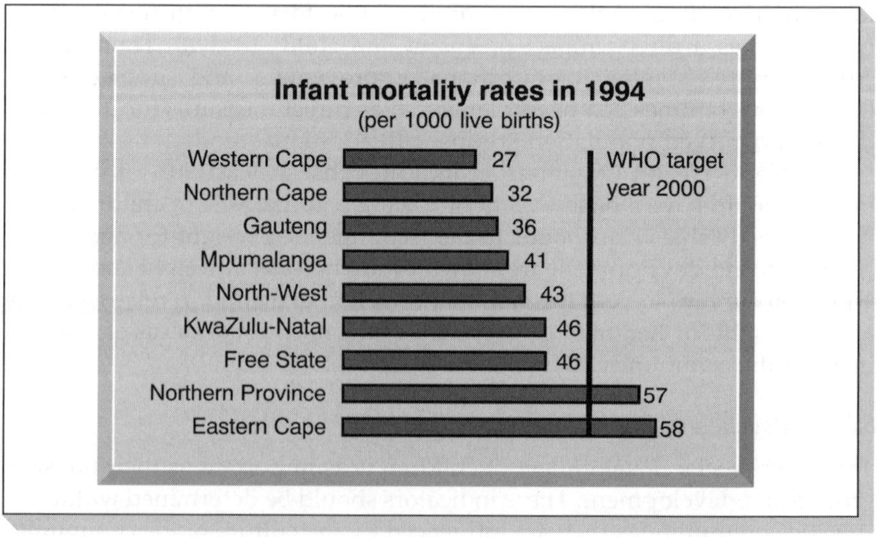

Source: Department of National Health and Population Development (1994)

- low birth weight of babies;
- attendance of baby clinics; and
- child minders.

8.3.4.4 The child and under-five mortality rate

The child mortality rate gives an indication of the number of deaths of children between the ages of one and four years in a given year per 1 000 children in that age group at the midpoint of the year. Child mortality excludes infant mortality while under-five mortality reflects both child and infant mortalities. The World Health Organisation (1987) reports that the child mortality can be 250 times higher in the less developed countries in comparison with the infant mortality.

8.3.4.5 Life expectancy at a given age

Life expectancy is an indicator of long-term survival and can also serve as an indicator of the general socio-economic status of a country. The life expectancy at birth is the average number of years lived by all those in the population concerned born alive. According to the World Health Organisation (1981:34), the ideal is that the life expectancy at birth should be over 60 years. The World Bank estimates that the life expectancy at birth for different income groups is:

- low-income countries - 61,1 years;
- low-middle-income countries - 64,0 years;
- high-middle-income countries - 67,3 years; and
- high-income countries - 76,1 years.

South Africa is classified as a middle-income country and has an average life expectancy of 64 years (South Africa (a) 1991:1).

8.3.4.6 Maternal mortality

Maternal mortality gives an indication of the risk of mothers during pregnancy and childbirth as well as the socio-economic conditions, the nutritional status and sanitation facilities in a specific community. It also serves as an indicator of the availability, accessibility and quality of health care. Maternal mortality is, however, strongly influenced by cultural norms and traditional practices. High parity, early and late child-bearing and short birth intervals are some of the factors that influence maternal health and maternal mortality. The maternal mortality rate is the number of deaths among women due to pregnancy and childbirth up to six weeks after delivery, expressed per live birth per year (South Africa (a) 1991).

Figure 8.3 illustrates the differences in maternal mortality rates in South Africa and other countries of various developmental levels.

FIGURE 8.2: Life expectancy comparisons (1985–1990)

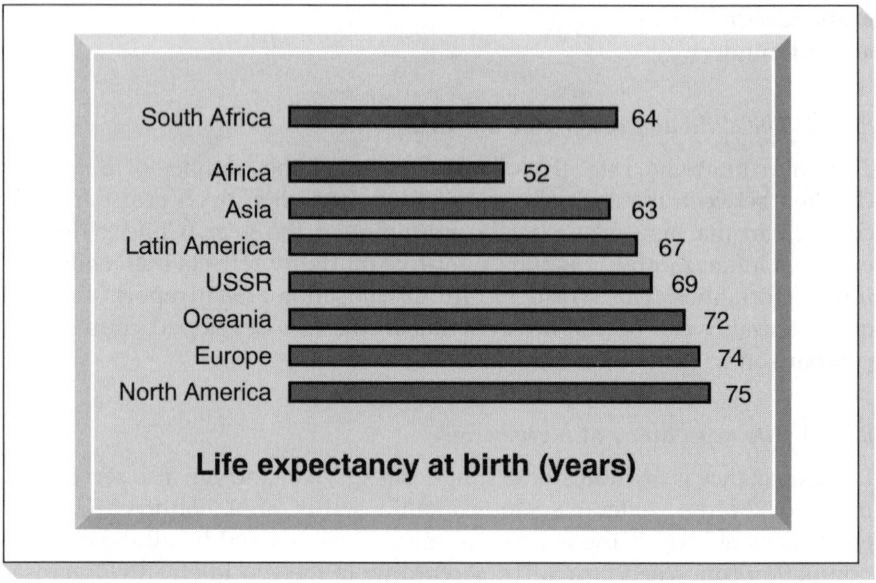

Source: Department of National Health and Population Development (1991b)

FIGURE 8.3: Maternal mortality rate comparison

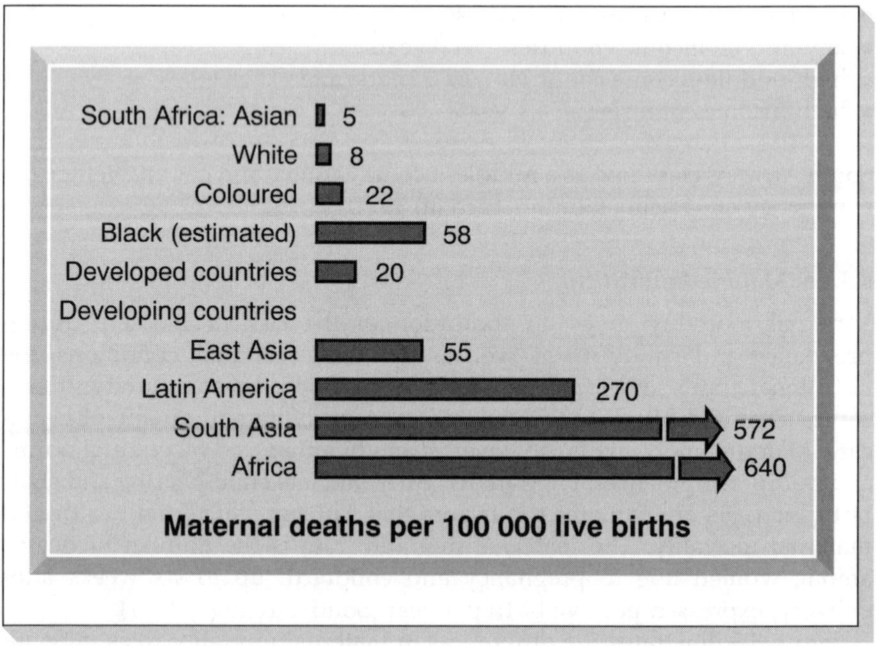

Source: Department of National Health and Population Development (1991a)

8.3.4.7 Disease-specific mortality and morbidity

Disease-specific mortality is calculated for specific causes of death. This includes specific causes for certain age groups and people of different socio-economic levels as well as for people living in certain geographical areas. Morbidity can be described as the incidence and/or prevalence of certain diseases or disabilities (WHO 1981:37). Morbidity rates usually reflect the six diseases most prevalent in a specific country, community or age group.

According to the World Health Organisation (1987:114), there has been a decline in the death rate from ischaemic heart diseases among younger men in several developed countries, but statistics show an increase in heart diseases in adults under 65 years of age. In some developing countries communicable diseases are still a major cause of mortality. Heart disease, however, is increasingly becoming a major problem in some of these countries due to the influence of westernisation and industrialisation.

Destructive life-styles associated with first-world living conditions, such as smoking-related diseases (for example, lung cancer), motor accidents, obesity, alcohol abuse, violence, homicide and suicide are no longer limited to the more affluent countries, but are becoming major problems in some developing countries as well.

Diseases such as malaria are still a major health problem in South Africa as well as in other regions. Tuberculosis, measles and some diarrhoea-related diseases remain a serious problem world-wide. In South Africa malaria continues to be a major health problem and due to the high rainfall and floods during 1996 the number of malaria cases increased dramatically. Tuberculosis is the most frequently notified disease in South Africa and a very serious health problem.

8.4 SELECTED GLOBAL INDICATORS

An international comparison on the health status of countries is very difficult. The World Health Organisation, in this regard, selected certain indicators for use at global level to make evaluation and monitoring possible for all countries. A limited number of indicators were selected from all the recommended indicators. Individual countries, however, may also use some of the other indicators to satisfy their own specific needs.

The following twelve indicators were selected:

- Health for all received endorsement as a policy at the highest official level.
- Mechanisms for involving people in the implementation of strategies have been formed and/or strengthened, and are actually functioning.
- At least 5% of the gross national product is spent on health.
- A reasonable percentage of the national health expenditure is devoted to local health care.
- Resources are equally distributed.

- The needs for external resources of a number of developing countries with well-defined strategies for health for all, accompanied by explicit resource allocations, are receiving sustained support from affluent countries.
- Primary health care is available to the whole population with at least the following:
  - immunisation against diphtheria, tetanus, whooping cough, measles, poliomyelitis and tuberculosis
  - local health care, including availability of at least 20 essential drugs, within one hour's walk or travel
  - safe water in the home or within 15 minutes' walking distance, and adequate sanitary facilities in the home or immediate vicinity
  - trained personnel for attending pregnancy and childbirth, and caring for children up to at least one year of age.
- The nutritional status of children is adequate, in that:
  - at least 90% of newborn infants have a birth weight of at least 2,5 kg
  - at least 90% of children have a weight-for-age corresponding to their height-for-age.
- The infant mortality rate for all identifiable subgroups is below 50 per 1 000 live births.
- Life expectancy at birth is over 60 years.
- The adult literacy rate for both men and women exceeds 70%.
- The gross national product per head exceeds US$500 (WHO 1981:39–40).

Due to the fact that the specified list of indicators was not comprehensive, the World Health Organisation recommended that all the member states be assisted in developing a system to test indicators in a district household survey. In September 1988 a list of twenty-seven indicators was tested through household surveys conducted according to specific guidelines by local personnel and community involvement. The main objective of this study was to test the validity of these indicators for monitoring progress towards health for all at district level, and to reformulate the indicators where applicable. Various recommendations were received from these countries for improvement and standardisation of the indicators.

South Africa also strives to comply with the aforementioned indicators but, as in many other developing countries, constraints such as unemployment, the rapidly increasing population, rapid urbanisation and declining living standards hamper progress.

The following ten important indicators were selected for South Africa:

- infant mortality;
- deaths under five (% of total deaths);
- teenage pregnancies (% of all pregnancies);
- HIV-incidence among pregnant women (%);
- the incidence of tuberculosis (per 100 000 of population);
- nutritional status;

FIGURE 8.4: The progress made from 1960–1990

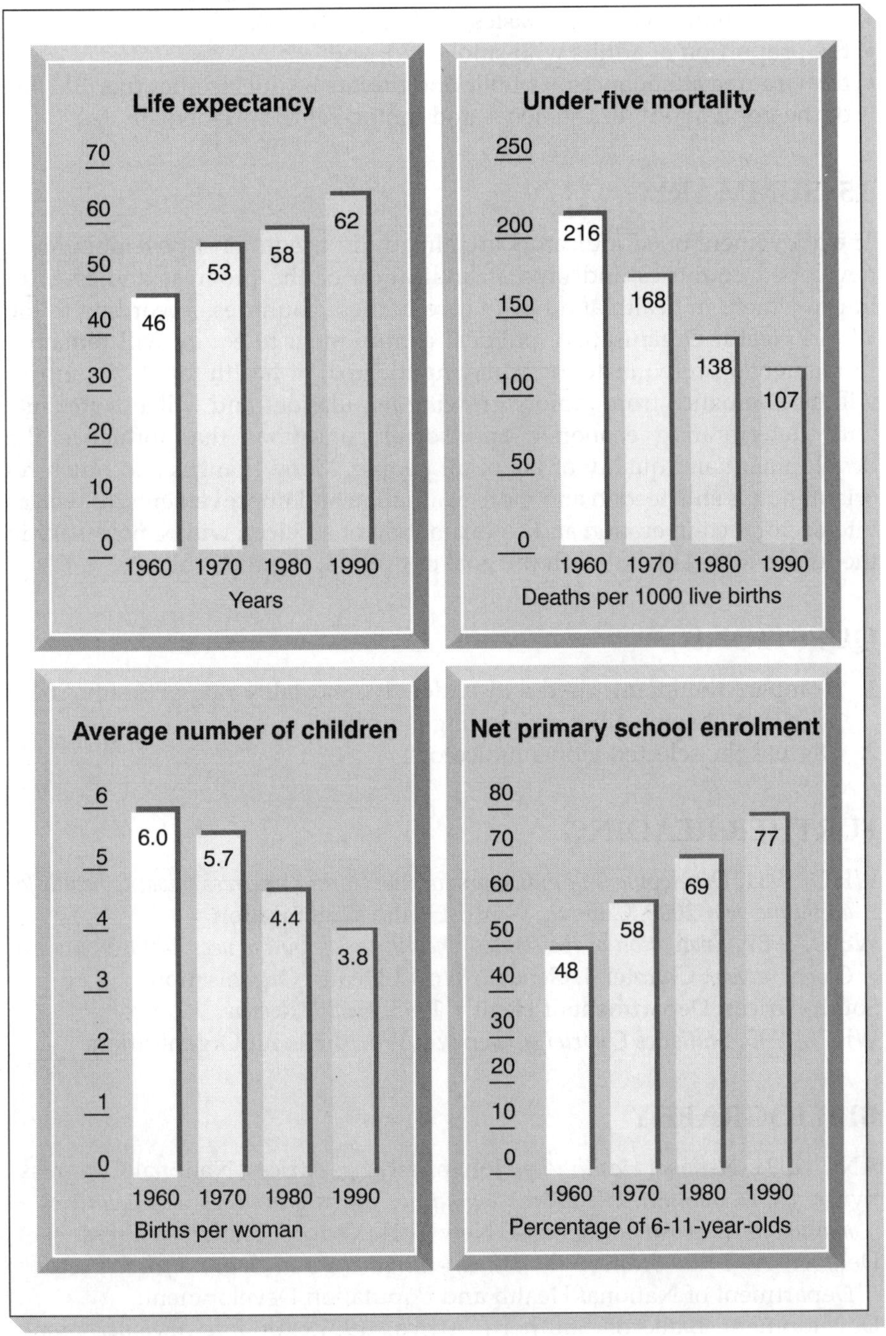

Source: Unicef (1995)

- low birth weight (% of all births);
- immunisation coverage (measles, DTP, polio, BCG);
- the proportion of adults who smoke (%); and
- total trauma attendances at public and private health facilities (per 100 000 of the population) (e.g. violence and motor-vehicle accidents).

8.5 SUMMARY

The abovementioned indicators are already in use in most developing and developed countries and give an indication of the progress and level of improvement in health and health care in these countries. According to the World Health Organisation, political commitment to equity will remain a fundamental prerequisite for achieving the goal of health for all. Countries will face demands from rapidly growing populations and will also struggle with deteriorating economic and social conditions that influence the development and quality of life of all people. Many changes and much re-orientation is still needed and more evaluation and improvements, as well as intersectoral co-operation and co-ordination of services, will be necessary in the future to be able to reach the goal of optimal health for all.

QUESTIONS

1. Compare the infant, child and under-five mortality rate of South Africa with that of some other developing countries.
2. Discuss the selected global indicators.

FURTHER READING

WHO. 1981. *Development of indicators for monitoring progress towards health for all by the year 2000.* Geneva: World Health Organisation.

WHO. 1987. *Evaluation of the strategy health for all by the year 2000. Volume 1. Global review.* Chapter 4. Geneva: World Health Organisation.

South African Department of Health. 1995. *Health Review.*

WHO. 1995. *Statistics Quarterly.* Geneva: World Health Organisation.

BIBLIOGRAPHY

ANC. 1994. *National Health Plan.* Johannesburg: African National Congress.

Byrne, M. & Bennett, F.J. 1986. *Community nursing in developing countries. A manual for the community nurse.* New York: Oxford University Press.

Delport, A. 1991. *Strategy for primary health care in South Africa.* Pretoria: Department of National Health and Population Development.

Development Bank of Southern Africa. 1991. *An inter-regional profile.* Midrand: Centre for Information Analysis.

South African Department of Health. 1995. *Health Review.*
South African Department of National Health and Population Development. 1988. *Health trends in South Africa.*
South African Department of National Health and Population Development. 1991a & 1994. *Health trends in South Africa.*
South African Department of National Health and Population Development. 1991b. *Annual report.*
Unicef. 1995. *The state of the world's children.* London: Oxford University Press.
WHO. 1995. *Statistics Quarterly.* Geneva: World Health Organisation.
WHO. 1981. *Development of indicators for monitoring progress towards health for all by the year 2000.* Geneva: World Health Organisation.
WHO. 1987. *Evaluation of the strategy health for all by the year 2000. Volume 1. Global review.* Geneva: World Health Organisation.

9 Marketing community health services

MARIE DREYER

CHAPTER OBJECTIVES

After reading this chapter, the student should be able to:

- introduce the concept of marketing health services;
- discuss appropriate marketing concepts;
- explain the role of the community nurse in respect of the marketing process.

9.1 INTRODUCTION

Marketing health care is a relatively new concept in the health-care industry and formal marketing has only recently became a functional area in health-care management. The marketing of health-care services is a difficult task because rendering health care is seen as a service and not as a business. Marketing techniques developed by the private sector may not be suitable for use in the public sector, but the basic concepts and principles are valid in any marketing situation. A successful programme for the purposes of marketing community nursing services will need skilful planning with careful attention to community attitudes and ethical issues.

9.2 THE MARKETING OF HEALTH CARE

A market can be described as a place where the transfer and trade of products, goods or services is negotiated. Wherever there is a potential for trade, a market could exist.

According to Hodgetts and Cascio (1983:348), marketing can be described as "the process of planning and managing all transactions between an organisation and its constituents". In the health-care field, the constituents are patients/clients, physicians, local communities and government agencies.

Marketing is defined by various experts in the business field and in most of these definitions the emphasis is on aspects such as planning, management, transactions, the product and consumers.

The marketing of health care is based on the principles and techniques developed by the private sector and is described by Sweeney, Berl and Winston (1989:4) as

> . . . an organised discipline for understanding: (1) how a health marketplace works; (2) the role in which the health organisation can render optimum services to the marketplace; (3) mechanisms for adjusting production capabilities for meeting consumer demand; and (4) how the organisation can assure patient satisfaction.

Picket and Hanlon (1990:244) see the marketing of health care as

> . . . a comprehensive programme involving the product of service, its cost, its distribution, and the education of the public to influence voluntary exchange transactions that will result in the prevention of disease and promotion of health.

Health care is first and foremost a service business and it requires a service-orientated approach to marketing. However, the contemporary health-care market is becoming increasingly an industry with a diverse set of buyers such as private practitioners, individuals or third parties who want to buy and sell products.

The products or goods of health care are services, facilities, surgical procedures, medicines, equipment and manpower training.

These products reach the market in the following ways:

- health care services are provided in exchange for financial payment;
- equipment is bought from providers by the health-care services; and
- medical schemes are offered to consumers of health care to assist them financially.

Furthermore, the health-care services look to the labour market for employees and use the financial market to obtain capital.

Tayson in Hein and Nicholson (1986:343) cites certain features that are common to both commercial and health-care products:

- The products are developed to fill a market need or want. In the case of a health care service, this need could be for physicians, hospitals or clinics.
- Capital is required for production, research and development of the product.
- Products must have specific functions or features and be packaged for maximum acceptance.
- Products are sold to selected market segments.

Various questions can be asked when marketing health care, such as:

- What kind of services do people want?
- Which trends may develop in future patient care?
- How will the health care organisation respond to new trends?

These questions should be addressed when a programme for marketing of health care is compiled.

It is important to determine the client's or patient's needs regarding health-care services as this will influence the kind of services that should be promoted when health care is marketed. Marketing managers should also be able to estimate future trends in patient care and the responses of health-care organisations to new trends. Throughout the marketing process, attention should be given to these aspects as the changing nature of health and disease influences the delivery of health care.

9.3 THE MARKETING PROCESS

The marketing process can be compared with the nursing process because both involve elements such as gathering and analysis of data, the determination of needs, planning and the development of strategies. In some marketing literature, managerial functions like policy, budgeting, organisation and control are emphasised. Functions that are highlighted here are marketing research, the marketing planning process, control and budgeting as well as certain key elements and concepts associated with marketing.

9.4 MARKETING RESEARCH

Marketing research or assessment is the first step to be taken before a product is marketed. This is essential for determining the needs, wants, expectations and demands of the potential buyers or consumers of a product. It also establishes the population that can be reached as well as opportunities, risks and trends in marketing.

This type of information helps marketing managers make better decisions. Marketing research and assessment are closely related and may result in the same type of information becoming available (Hillestad & Berkowitz 1984).

Effective research involves an outline of the goal or reasons for undertaking research, as well as the selection of appropriate methods or tools to gather data, the analysis and interpretation of the data and the presentation of the findings. Whenever research is conducted, these steps of the research process must be followed to be sure that relevant data are collected.

The marketing research function consists of the collection and analysis of data on the environment from the health-care organisation. The environment includes aspects such as the positive and negative points of the organisation, suppliers, customers, competition and other factors that may affect the marketing of the specific service. It also includes data in relation to certain uncontrollable factors such as economic conditions, demographic and social/cultural changes, political and legal constraints and technical development. Marketing research provides an ongoing basis for data collection and feedback.

The research process can also serve as an evaluation instrument to evaluate risks, consumer satisfaction, marketing demands and the growth of the market.

The marketing audit is one method that can be used to examine and evaluate the marketing environment, objectives, strategies and activities of an organisation with a view to determining problem areas and to making recommendations. During the audit, specific lists of primary and secondary targets can be made that will consist of those communities that can be served best.

The audit is an organised effort to monitor, assess and judge the quality of care, the consumer satisfaction or the appropriateness of strategies.

Marketing research is of great importance and its value must not be underestimated. The data or research results provide the basis for decision-making when marketing a product. Proper analysis and interpretation of the findings lay the foundation for the marketing-planning process.

9.5 THE MARKETING-PLANNING PROCESS

This is the next important step after the research is completed. The principles for the development of a marketing programme are similar to those of a health-care plan but in this case a more market-orientated approach is necessary. The planning of the marketing programme is based on the research results, and priorities, goals and objectives are set accordingly. Marketing goals outline the general results desired outcomes, while objectives define the specific, measurable outcomes that can be achieved.

During the planning process the needs, demands and preferences of the consumers of health care must be understood, and their views of what is important in their lives and for their health should be considered.

A further essential aspect in marketing health care services is the establishment of a marketing committee that consists of experts in the field of marketing as well as leaders in the health-care field. The main function of this committee is to take care of certain complex tasks such as the development of proper relations between marketing planners and providers of health care, staff members and the media.

This committee can be responsible for the co-ordination of all the functions of the marketing planners.

Important factors to consider in the planning process are the policies, marketing philosophy and the specific mission of the organisation.

Specific marketing policies provide guidelines and direction in decision-making and should be in line with the marketing objectives. Policies for marketing health care must be flexible, consistent, objective and acceptable to those who must apply them. All the individuals who have to apply the policies must be well informed and everyone joining an organisation should be familiar with the relevant policies.

The formulation of a marketing philosophy and mission is important, as this will reflect the values and beliefs that could direct the approach towards marketing, especially in the case of marketing health care. The philosophy of

FIGURE 9.1: The marketing-planning process

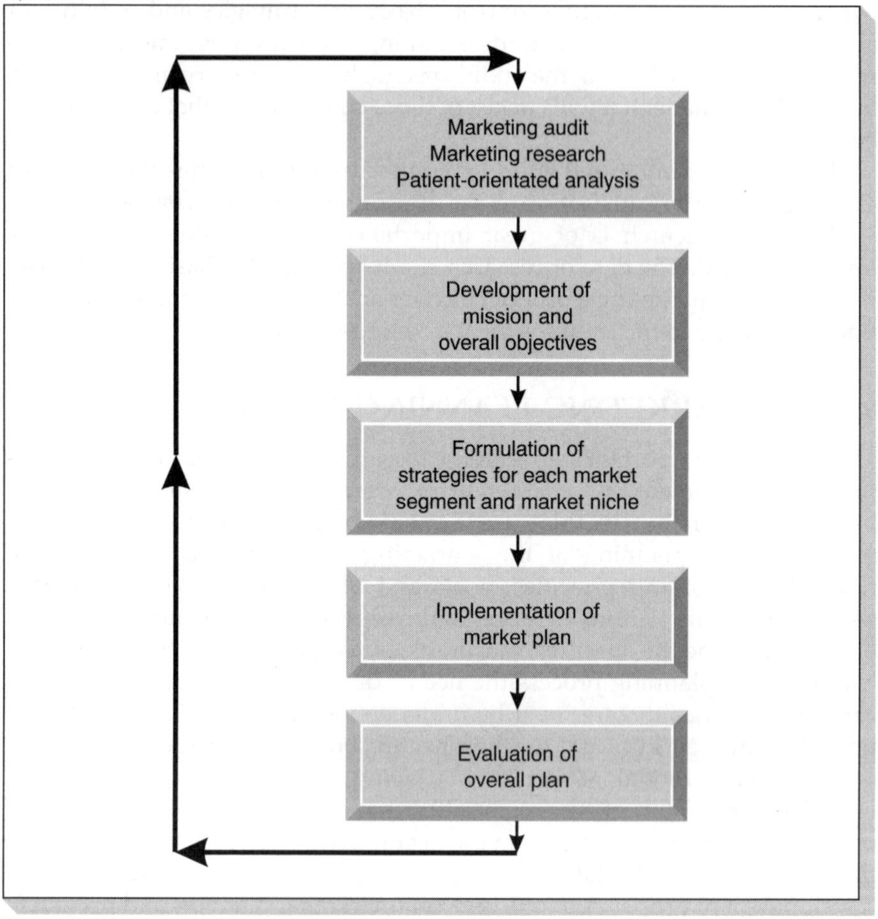

Source: Hodgetts & Cascio (1983)

an organisation determines the quality of the service or product to be delivered as well as the attitudes towards other people and their values and beliefs.

Certain key elements should also be considered in a marketing plan, i.e. segments, product, price, place and promotion.

The segments are specific sections of a target population with a specific need or interest. A population is broken down into segments to make it easier to develop strategies for priority groups. A segment may be classified as follows:

- *Demographic segments:* These refer to age, race and sex characteristics.
- *Geographic segments:* These refer to location, neighbourhoods, work place, etc.

- *Psychographic segments:* These include life-styles, attitudes and behaviour patterns.

The products or services are made available to the target population at a place such as a hospital, clinic or outpatient department, with the product being either a service, a health-promotion programme or an audiovisual aid. The product should be designed to provide the population with a desired benefit such as learning a new skill or solving a health problem (Edelman & Mandle 1990:180). If the product is the promotion of health through health education, the target group should be aware that it is available and where and when it is obtainable. This includes the methods and techniques used by the organisation to let people know about the service. The price refers to the fees paid by consumers for services rendered, which are sometimes determined by the government, insurance companies or private organisations.

Other marketing concepts of great importance that should be considered during the planning process are profitability, consumer orientation, community responsibility and co-operation. In the case of profitability the

FIGURE 9.2: Elements of health-care marketing

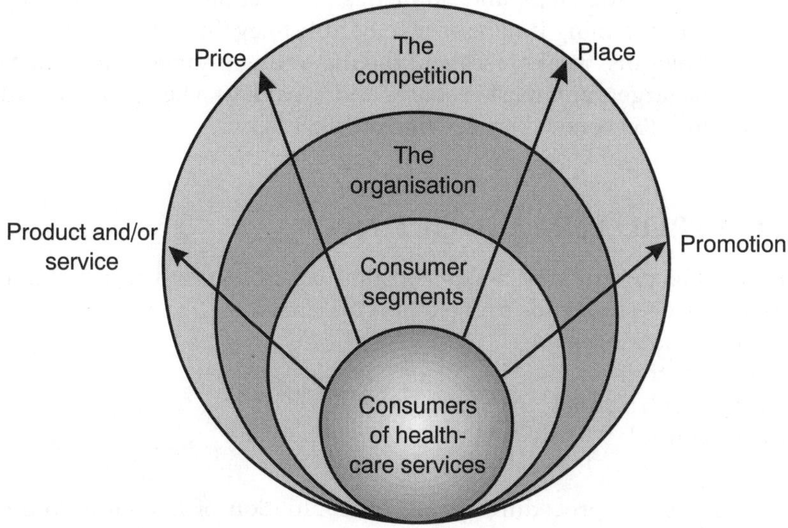

Source: Hodgetts & Cascio (1983)

questions to be asked could be: What does a health service gain from marketing health care? Is it financial gain or improvement of the health status of the community, or both? In the case of a private health service, making a profit can be of great importance, but in the case of a public health service it is more important to render a service to the community.

Consumer orientation means that the needs of the consumer of health care should be considered. When marketing a health-care service, the community as well as the authorities responsible for health care must be involved and the marketing manager should adhere to the relevant legislation and regulations. Co-operation between the target community and providers of health care is essential for success.

With the philosophy and specific mission in mind, marketing strategies and tactics are selected and developed. When strategies are developed, aspects such as the price, product, place and promotion should be considered. A strategy may, for example, be the decision to advertise to a certain target group with the tactics describing the type of advertisement, the size and colour or the location. Marketing strategies are, however, much more than advertising. They require a careful plan with consistent action (Picket & Hanlon 1990:35).

A strategic plan is important because it provides a direction for an organisation as well as a specific point at which the marketing function can start. A formal written marketing plan, which forms the framework for the layout of the specific steps and strategies, is essential for any marketing process. Proper planning is necessary to be able to evaluate the marketplace, to identify strengths, weaknesses and the marketing segments, as well as to determine the targets and market shares and to achieve a key position within the community (Sweeney, Berl & Winston 1989:11).

9.6 CONTROL AND BUDGETING

The marketing programme needs constant control to ensure profitability. The control process extends to the following areas:

- annual evaluation;
- financial control;
- efficiency control; and
- strategic control.

The annual control procedures entail an evaluation of the sales volumes, market shares, profit margins and sales expenses. They also include the development of a marketing budget, the implementation time-line, organisational charts and a control system. The time-line gives an outline of the dates and time for planning, implementation and control phases, while the organisational chart indicates the lines of authority.

The control system measures the performance of the marketing programme against the goals and objectives that were formulated during the planning phase.

The health-care organisation should review and analyse market shares, costs, profit and sales on a regular basis, while also monitoring the cost-effectiveness of marketing strategies and tactics used for the purpose of marketing health care. The costs of marketing a health service product involve more than money. The value exchange must be acceptable and affordable to the target population. The price of the health-service product is of great importance because if the price is too low the consumers may think that the service is not valuable enough. Thus the question is often: What are people willing to pay and how much can they afford?

Annual budgeting is necessary to make provision for funds that can be utilised for marketing purposes. The budget is a tool used for planning as well as control; it is linked to the objectives of the organisation and it forecasts the direct and indirect expenses in respect of the development, implementation and control of the marketing plan.

According to Sweeney, Berl and Winston (1989:431), the budgeting process for marketing health care is a complex and detailed procedure, which comprises revenues and expenses under the control of a specific marketing department.

9.7 GENERAL CONSIDERATIONS AND CONSTRAINTS

A number of problems and constraints have been identified in the marketing of community health care that render the application of the private sector's marketing strategies and techniques difficult. Some of these are listed below:

- Community health care has many objectives such as: protecting workers, cleaning up the environment and preventing teenage pregnancy.
- Health care is a service and cannot be transferred to another owner, stored and recalled for later use or transported.
- Non-profit organisations are not willing to market what they believe to be an essential service.
- The managers of health services are usually people who are not trained in and have little experience of marketing, while physicians filling these posts often discourage marketing as unprofessional because of its promotional goal.
- Conflicting messages in the advertising of preventative or promotive health care may confuse the consumer.
- Health promotion often involves choices and changes that are not acceptable to the specific target group.
- Many health promotion and/or disease prevention advertisements focus on an entire population rather than on a specific segment with a specific need. A segment may have geographic, socio-economic or demographic

features that render it distinct from other segments and this results in different responses.
- Dishonesty in marketing programmes will not be tolerated by any organisation or consumer of the service. For example, if the sponsors promise to deliver a certain product but are unable to do so, the programme will fail.
- The image of the government or agency will have an impact on the marketing programme - distrust or a negative image will have an influence on the acceptability of a programme.
- The ongoing changes, new approaches and strategies in the provision of health care complicate the marketing of health care.

These constraints may hamper the marketing of community health care, particularly as health care is viewed as an essential service. It is therefore important that specific strategies and tactics be developed to market health care. The approach should be service orientated and acceptable to the consumers of health care as this will have an influence on their loyalty towards the services offered. The community nurse who is part of the community health-care service product must take cognisance of these constraints. She must be able to provide a service of such high quality that the service markets itself. The way in which the needs of the clients are met, gives one service a "competitive edge over another" (Hein & Nicholson 1986:345).

9.8 THE ROLE OF THE COMMUNITY NURSE IN THE PROVISION OF A MARKET-ORIENTATED SERVICE

As provider of community health care, the community nurse must realise that the health service market is competitive and that she must play an active and leading role in the promotion of community health services. Health-care services must be acceptable, affordable and accessible, otherwise consumers will look for other health-care resources to satisfy their health-care needs. Community leaders should at all times be involved in the development of marketing procedures and strategies because they understand their own people and would know what kind of advertisement would be acceptable and could motivate people to use an advertised service or product. Members of the community must be involved and encouraged to participate in the planning and provision of health care as well as in marketing these services. To be able to participate in marketing, the target population must be aware of the product and its benefit to them. Public relations, advertising strategies and sales approaches are of great importance in getting the co-operation of the community - the selected strategies or advertising messages chosen should reach the people.

The community nurse must formulate specific short- and long-term objectives, which should be realistic and attainable. She must also provide the necessary information to the public regarding the available services and the goals and objectives of these services. Through the provision of quality care, the proper utilisation of resources, the acknowledgement of the consumer as a partner, and through informing and teaching the community, marketing of community health-care services can take place.

Marketing is important and brings health care to the attention of consumers - not only in profit-orientated services but also in non-profit institutions. Community nurses can play an important role in a health-service marketing programme because they form a very large part of the health personnel and can generate consumer satisfaction through the provision of quality nursing care.

Marketing can be applied in any organisation and must be sensitive to consumer needs. However, a balance between what consumers think they need and what they really need should be maintained. Frequently the priorities set by the community health personnel do not meet the needs of the consumers. It is essential to keep in mind that the approach in marketing health care should be service orientated.

9.9 SUMMARY

In this chapter an outline is given of the aspects related to marketing in general and the application of some of these principles in marketing community health-care services. Various constraints in marketing health care and the application of marketing principles are listed and the role and functions of the community nurse are discussed. The importance of a service-orientated approach in the marketing of health-care services cannot be overemphasised, as this will influence the attitudes and loyalty of the consumers of health-care services. The community nurse may play a vital role in the marketing process because of her close contact with the clients or consumers. Her competence and expertise and the way in which she organises and provides community health care can be an advertisement for the product. The business of community health-care delivery is mainly the promotion of health and the prevention of disease, and this should be emphasised in the marketing process.

QUESTIONS

1. Discuss the principles involved in marketing a health-care service.
2. What is meant by "segmentation"?
3. What are the most important constraints in marketing a health service?
4. Write short notes on the various elements that should be addressed in the marketing plan.

FURTHER READING

Hodgetts, R.M. & Cascio, D.M. 1983. *Modern health care administration.* Chapter 16. New York: Academic Press.

Picket, G. & Hanlon, J.J. 1990. *Public health administration and practice.* Chapter 12. St Louis: Mosby.

BIBLIOGRAPHY

Edelman, C.L. & Mandle, C.L. 1990. *Health promotion through the life-span.* St Louis: Mosby.

Hein, E.C. & Nicholson, M.J. 1986. *Contemporary leadership behaviour: selected readings.* Boston: Little Brown & Company.

Hillestad, S.G. & Berkowitz, E.N. 1984. *Health care marketing plans: from strategy to action.* Glenview, Illinois: Dow Jones-Irwin.

Hodgetts, R.M. & Cascio, D.M. 1983. *Modern health care administration.* New York: Academic Press.

Picket, G. & Hanlon, J.J. 1990. *Public health administration and practice.* St Louis: Mosby.

Sweeney, R.E., Berl, R. & Winston, W.J. 1989. *Cases and select readings in health care marketing.* New York: The Haworth Press.

Index

Other Nursing and/or Community Nursing titles published by International Thomson Publishing Southern Africa (Pty) Ltd:

Series: *Community Health Care in Southern Africa*

Dennill, King, Lock & Swanepoel, *Aspects of Primary Health Care*, 1995
(ISBN: 1-86864-081-7)

Bouwer, Dreyer, Herselman, Lock & Zeelie, *Contemporary Trends in Community Nursing*, 1997
(ISBN: 1-86864-009-4)

Hattingh, Van der Merwe, Van Rensburg & Dreyer, *Gerontology*, 1996
(ISBN: 1-86864-008-6)

Other:

Jooste & Troskie, *Staff Development for Nurses*, 1995
(ISBN: 1-86812-510-6)

Where to purchase these books

The above titles are available from your local academic bookseller or contact us directly for further details.

ORDERS

International Thomson Publishing Southern Africa (Pty) Ltd
P.O. Box 2459
Halfway House
1685

Tel: (011) 805-4819
Fax: (011) 805-3648

MAILING LIST

If you wish to be added to our mailing list, please send the following information to the above address:

Full name and address (including postal code)
Telephone number and, if available, fax number and e-mail address